Modern Approach to the Salivary Glands

Editors

M. BOYD GILLESPIE
WILLIAM R. RYAN

OTOLARYNGOLOGIC CLINICS OF NORTH AMERICA

www.oto.theclinics.com

Consulting Editor
SUJANA S. CHANDRASEKHAR

June 2021 • Volume 54 • Number 3

ELSEVIER

1600 John F. Kennedy Boulevard • Suite 1800 • Philadelphia, Pennsylvania, 19103-2899

http://www.oto.theclinics.com

OTOLARYNGOLOGIC CLINICS OF NORTH AMERICA Volume 54, Number 3
June 2021 ISSN 0030-6665, ISBN-13: 978-0-323-81331-0

Editor: Stacy Eastman
Developmental Editor: Diana Ang

Photocopying

Single photocopies of single articles may be made for personal use as allowed by national copyright laws. Permission of the Publisher and payment of a fee is required for all other photocopying, including multiple or systematic copying, copying for advertising or promotional purposes, resale, and all forms of document delivery. Special rates are available for educational institutions that wish to make photocopies for non-profit educational classroom use. For information on how to seek permission visit www.elsevier.com/permissions or call: (+44) 1865 843830 (UK)/(+1) 215 239 3804 (USA).

Derivative Works

Subscribers may reproduce tables of contents or prepare lists of articles including abstracts for internal circulation within their institutions. Permission of the Publisher is required for resale or distribution outside the institution. Permission of the Publisher is required for all other derivative works, including compilations and translations (please consult www.elsevier.com/permissions).

Electronic Storage or Usage

Permission of the Publisher is required to store or use electronically any material contained in this periodical, including any article or part of an article (please consult www.elsevier.com/permissions). Except as outlined above, no part of this publication may be reproduced, stored in a retrieval system or transmitted in any form or by any means, electronic, mechanical, photocopying, recording or otherwise, without prior written permission of the Publisher.

Notice

No responsibility is assumed by the Publisher for any injury and/or damage to persons or property as a matter of products liability, negligence or otherwise, or from any use or operation of any methods, products, instructions or ideas contained in the material herein. Because of rapid advances in the medical sciences, in particular, independent verification of diagnoses and drug dosages should be made.

Although all advertising material is expected to conform to ethical (medical) standards, inclusion in this publication does not constitute a guarantee or endorsement of the quality or value of such product or of the claims made of it by its manufacturer.

Otolaryngologic Clinics of North America (ISSN 0030-6665) is published bimonthly by Elsevier, Inc., 360 Park Avenue South, New York, NY 10010-1710. Months of issue are February, April, June, August, October, and December. Business and Editorial Offices: 1600 John F. Kennedy Blvd., Suite 1800, Philadelphia, PA 19103-2899. Customer Service Office: 6277 Sea Harbor Drive, Orlando, FL 32887-4800. Periodicals postage paid at New York, NY and additional mailing offices. Subscription prices are $437.00 per year (US individuals), $1278.00 per year (US institutions), $100.00 per year (US & Canadian student/resident), $559.00 per year (Canadian individuals), $1348.00 per year (Canadian institutions), $610.00 per year (international individuals), $1348.00 per year (international institutions), $270.00 per year (international student/resident). Foreign air speed delivery is included in all *Clinics'* subscription prices. All prices are subject to change without notice. **POSTMASTER:** Send address changes to *Otolaryngologic Clinics of North America*, Elsevier Health Sciences Division, Subscription Customer Service, 3251 Riverport Lane, Maryland Heights, MO 63043. **Telephone: 1-800-654-2452 (U.S. and Canada); 314-447-8871 (outside U.S. and Canada). Fax: 314-447-8029. E-mail: journalscustomerservice-usa@elsevier.com (for print support); journalsonlinesupport-usa@elsevier.com (for online support).**

Reprints. For copies of 100 or more of articles in this publication, please contact the Commercial Reprints Department, Elsevier Inc., 360 Park Avenue South, New York, NY 10010-1710. Tel.: 212-633-3874; Fax: 212-633-3820; E-mail: reprints@elsevier.com.

Otolaryngologic Clinics of North America is also published in Spanish by McGraw-Hill Interamericana Editores S.A., P.O. Box 5-237, 06500 Mexico D.F., Mexico.

Otolaryngologic Clinics of North America is covered in *MEDLINE/PubMed (Index Medicus), Current Contents/Clinical Medicine, Excerpta Medica, BIOSIS, Science Citation Index,* and *ISI/BIOMED.*

Contributors

CONSULTING EDITOR

SUJANA S. CHANDRASEKHAR, MD, FACS, FAAOHNS
Past President, American Academy of Otolaryngology–Head and Neck Surgery, Secretary-Treasurer, American Otological Society, Partner, ENT & Allergy Associates, LLP, Clinical Professor, Department of Otolaryngology–Head and Neck Surgery, Zucker School of Medicine at Hofstra-Northwell, Hempstead, New York; Clinical Associate Professor, Department of Otolaryngology–Head and Neck Surgery, Icahn School of Medicine at Mount Sinai, New York, New York

EDITORS

M. BOYD GILLESPIE, MD, MSc
Professor and Chair, Department of Otolaryngology–Head and Neck Surgery, University of Tennessee Health Science Center, Memphis, Tennessee

WILLIAM R. RYAN, MD, FACS
Associate Professor, Head and Neck Oncologic, Endocrine, and Salivary Surgery, Department of Otolaryngology–Head and Neck Surgery, University of California, San Francisco, San Francisco, California

JENNIFER A. VILLWOCK, MD
Department of Otolaryngology–Head and Neck Surgery, Kansas University, University of Kansas Medical Center, Kansas City, Kansas

AUTHORS

CHRISTOPHER D. BADGER, MD, MBA
Division of Otolaryngology–Head and Neck Surgery, George Washington University School of Medicine & Health Sciences, Washington, DC

SOLY BAREDES, MD, FACS
Department of Otolaryngology–Head and Neck Surgery, Center for Skull Base and Pituitary Surgery, Neurological Institute of New Jersey, Rutgers New Jersey Medical School, Newark, New Jersey

GREGORY L. BARINSKY, PharmD
Department of Otolaryngology–Head and Neck Surgery, Rutgers New Jersey Medical School, Newark, New Jersey

DANIEL A. BENITO, MD
Division of Otolaryngology–Head and Neck Surgery, George Washington University School of Medicine & Health Sciences, Washington, DC

EVE M. R. BOWERS, BA
Department of Otolaryngology, University of Pittsburgh Medical Center, Medical Student, University of Pittsburgh School of Medicine, Pittsburgh, Pennsylvania.

DAVID J. BROWN, MD
Department of Otolaryngology–Head and Neck Surgery, Michigan Medicine, Ann Arbor, Michigan

CRISTINA CABRERA-MUFFLY, MD
Department of Otolaryngology–Head and Neck Surgery, University of Colorado School of Medicine, Aurora, Colorado

SUJANA S. CHANDRASEKHAR, MD, FACS, FAAOHNS
Past President, American Academy of Otolaryngology–Head and Neck Surgery, Secretary-Treasurer, American Otological Society, Partner, ENT & Allergy Associates, LLP, Clinical Professor, Department of Otolaryngology–Head and Neck Surgery, Zucker School of Medicine at Hofstra-Northwell, Hempstead, New York; Clinical Associate Professor, Department of Otolaryngology–Head and Neck Surgery, Icahn School of Medicine at Mount Sinai, New York, New York

JOLIE L. CHANG, MD, FACS
Associate Professor, Department of Otolaryngology–Head and Neck Surgery, University of California, San Francisco, San Francisco, California

C. ALESSANDRA COLAIANNI, MD
Instructor, Department of Otolaryngology-Head and Neck Surgery, Vanderbilt University Medical Center, Nashville, Tennessee

ANDREW B. DAVIS, MD
Otolaryngology Department, University of Iowa Hospitals and Clinics, Iowa City, Iowa

JEAN ANDERSON ELOY, MD, FARS, FACS
Chairman and Chief of Service, Department of Otolaryngology and Facial Plastic Surgery, Saint Barnabas Medical Center - RWJBarnabas Health, Livingston; Professor and Vice Chairman, Director, Rhinology and Sinus Surgery, Director, Otolaryngology Research, Co-Director, Endoscopic Skull Base Surgery Program, Department of Otolaryngology–Head and Neck Surgery, Professor of Neurological Surgery, Professor of Ophthalmology and Visual Science, Neurological Institute of New Jersey, Rutgers New Jersey Medical School, Newark, New Jersey

BRANDON I. ESIANOR, MD
Department of Otolaryngology–Head and Neck Surgery, Vanderbilt University Medical Center, Nashville, Tennessee

CHRISTINA H. FANG, MD
Rhinology, Sinus, and Endoscopic Skull Base Surgery Fellow, Department of Otolaryngology–Head and Neck Surgery, Rutgers New Jersey Medical School, Newark, New Jersey

M. BOYD GILLESPIE, MD, MSc
Professor and Chair, Department of Otolaryngology–Head and Neck Surgery, University of Tennessee Health Science Center, Memphis, Tennessee

STACEY T. GRAY, MD, FARS, FACS
Associate Professor and Vice Chair of Otolaryngology Education, Residency Program Director Department of Otolaryngology–Head and Neck Surgery, Harvard Medical

School, Department of Otolaryngology–Head and Neck Surgery, Massachusetts Eye and Ear, Boston, Massachusetts

PATRICK K. HA, MD
Department of Otolaryngology–Head and Neck Surgery, University of California, San Francisco, San Francisco, California

TREVOR HACKMAN, MD, FACS
Department of Otolaryngology–Head and Neck Surgery, The University of North Carolina at Chapel Hill, UNC Hospitals, Chapel Hill, North Carolina

BRIANNA N. HARRIS, MD
Department of Otolaryngology–Head and Neck Surgery, Scripps Health

HENRY T. HOFFMAN, MD
Otolaryngology Department, University of Iowa Hospitals and Clinics, Iowa City, Iowa

ARJUN S. JOSHI, MD
Division of Otolaryngology–Head and Neck Surgery, George Washington University School of Medicine & Health Sciences, Washington, DC

HYUNSEOK KANG, MD
Department of Hematology and Oncology, University of California, San Francisco, San Francisco, California

ALEXANDRA E. KEJNER, MD, FACS
Department of Otolaryngology–Head and Neck Surgery, University of Kentucky, Lexington, Kentucky

NICOLE KLOOSTERMAN, BS
Vanderbilt University School of Medicine, Nashville, Tennessee

DENNIS KRAUS, MD, FACS
Department of Otolaryngology–Head and Neck Surgery, Lenox Hill Hospital Affiliated to the Zucker School of Medicine at Hofstra University

ANDREW R. LARSON, MD
Department of Otolaryngology–Head and Neck Surgery, Massachusetts Eye and Ear, Harvard Medical School, Boston, Massachusetts

MYRIAM LOYO, MD, MCR
Department of Otolaryngology, Oregon Health and Sciences University, Portland, Oregon

JENNIFER MOY, MD
Department of Otolaryngology, Oregon Health and Sciences University, Portland, Oregon

M. ALLISON OGDEN, MD, FACS
Department of Otolaryngology–Head and Neck Surgery, Washington University School of Medicine, St Louis, Missouri

NEELAM PRAKASH PHALKE, MD
Resident, Department of Otolaryngology–Head and Neck Surgery, Louisiana State University Health Sciences Campus, New Orleans, Louisiana

JANYN QUIZ, BS
Department of Otolaryngology–Head and Neck Surgery, University of Tennessee Health Science Center, Memphis, Tennessee

LEIGHTON F. REED, MD
Department of Otolaryngology–Head and Neck Surgery, University of Tennessee Health Science Center, Memphis, Tennessee

JEREMY D. RICHMON, MD
Associate Professor, Department of Otolaryngology-Head & Neck Surgery, Harvard Medical School, Massachusetts Eye and Ear, Boston, Massachusetts

BARAK RINGEL, MD
Department of Otolaryngology–Head and Neck Surgery, Lenox Hill Hospital Affiliated to the Zucker School of Medicine at Hofstra University

WILLIAM R. RYAN, MD, FACS
Associate Professor, Head and Neck Oncologic, Endocrine, and Salivary Surgery, Department of Otolaryngology–Head and Neck Surgery, University of California, San Francisco, San Francisco, California

MIRABELLE SAJISEVI, MD
Assistant Professor, Department of Surgery, Division of Otolaryngology, University of Vermont Medical Center, Burlington, Vermont

BARRY SCHAITKIN, MD
Professor, Department of Otolaryngology, University of Pittsburgh Medical Center, Shadyside Hospital, Pittsburgh, Pennsylvania

S. ANDREW SKILLINGTON, MD, MSCI
Department of Otolaryngology–Head and Neck Surgery, Washington University School of Medicine, St Louis, Missouri

KIMBERLY N. VINSON, MD
Department of Otolaryngology–Head and Neck Surgery, Vanderbilt University Medical Center, Nashville, Tennessee

KATHERINE C. WAI, MD
Department of Otolaryngology–Head and Neck Surgery, University of California, San Francisco, San Francisco, California

ROHAN WALVEKAR, MD
Mervin L. Trail Endowed Chair in Head and Neck Oncology, Department of Otolaryngology–Head and Neck Surgery, Louisiana State University Health Sciences Campus, New Orleans, Louisiana

MARK K. WAX, MD, FRCS(C)
Department of Otolaryngology, Oregon Health and Sciences University, Portland, Oregon

MARY JUE XU, MD
Department of Otolaryngology–Head and Neck Surgery, University of California, San Francisco, San Francisco, California

Contents

Foreword: Salivary Gland Disease: A Comprehensive Resource   xiii

Sujana S. Chandrasekhar

Preface: The Science and Art of Salivary Care   xv

M. Boyd Gillespie and William R. Ryan

Basics

Practical Salivary Ultrasound Imaging Tips and Pearls   471

Mary Jue Xu and Jolie L. Chang

Ultrasound imaging is a valuable and effective clinical tool for salivary gland disorder evaluation and management. Pathologies including salivary duct stenosis, sialolithiasis, neoplasms, and autoimmune disorders have characteristic sonographic features. Maneuvers such as bimanual palpation and oral administration of sialagogues during the ultrasound examination can enhance examination findings. Ultrasound guidance is useful for targeting needle biopsies of neoplasms, ensuring appropriate intraparenchymal gland injections, and augmenting salivary duct instrumentation and intraoperative management.

Indications for Facial Nerve Monitoring During Parotidectomy   489

Mirabelle Sajisevi

Facial nerve injury is the most feared complication during parotid surgery. Intraoperative electromyographic nerve monitoring can be used to identify the facial nerve, map its course, identify surgical maneuvers detrimental to the nerve, and provide prognostic information. Multiple studies corroborate lower incidence of transient weakness in primary parotidectomy. In contrast, the incidence of permanent weakness has not been shown to be significantly affected by use of nerve monitoring. For revision surgery, studies show that monitored patients had (1) weakness that was less severe with quicker recovery and (2) shorter operative times compared with unmonitored patients.

IgG4-Related Disease and the Salivary Glands: A Review of Pathophysiology, Diagnosis, and Management   497

S. Andrew Skillington and M. Allison Ogden

IgG4-related disease is a rare, immune-mediated, systemic disease that is characterized by soft tissue lymphocyte infiltration and resultant fibrosis. The salivary glands are among the most commonly affected organs. Patients present with subacute submandibular and/or parotid swelling and sialadenitis. Diagnosis incorporates clinical, serologic, radiologic, and pathologic findings. Most cases respond quickly to systemic glucocorticoids. IgG4-related disease mimics many infectious, inflammatory, and neoplastic diseases. Therefore, IgG4-related disease is frequently misdiagnosed. A knowledge of the pathophysiology, diagnosis, and management of IgG4-related disease is important for providers who treat salivary gland diseases.

Surgical Techniques

Incorporating Sialendoscopy into the Otolaryngology Clinic   509

Christopher D. Badger, Daniel A. Benito, and Arjun S. Joshi

Simple sialendoscopy procedures may be performed in the outpatient clinic with few complications. This process spares patients the risks, increased cost, and time burdens of sialendoscopy under general anesthesia. Sialendoscopy procedures may be incorporated into the outpatient practice after gaining experience with these procedures in the operating room. Diagnostic sialendoscopy, dilation of stenosis, and endoscopic sialolithotomies of small, freely mobile stones are appropriate for in-office sialendoscopy in many instances.

Open Approaches to Stensen Duct Scar   521

Leighton F. Reed, M. Boyd Gillespie, and Trevor Hackman

Duct scar in the form of stenoses or stricture is the second leading cause of obstructive sialadenitis after stone. Over the past decade, there has been a growing experience demonstrating the effectiveness of endoscopic techniques in the minimally invasive management of salivary duct stenosis. Less information, however, is available with regard to open approaches for recurrent or complex ductal stenoses. This article reports on a case of gland preservation using an open ductal technique that originally was applied in cases of traumatic Stensen's duct injury.

Transoral Excision of Parapharyngeal Space Tumors   531

Andrew R. Larson and William R. Ryan

Transoral excision of parapharyngeal space (PPS) tumors has increased in popularity along with the increased use of robotic and endoscopic surgical technology. Here, the authors highlight the indications, techniques, outcomes, and complications of transoral approaches to PPS tumors, with a special emphasis on salivary tumors of the PPS and the transoral robotic surgery approach.

Management of Mucoceles, Sialoceles, and Ranulas   543

Eve M.R. Bowers and Barry Schaitkin

Mucoceles are common salivary gland disorders. Mucoceles are benign, mucus-filled extravasation pseudocysts that commonly arise on the lower lip of children and young adults. Although surgical excision is commonly performed to remove these lesions, other treatments include marsupialization, micromarsupialization laser ablation, cryotherapy, intralesional steroid injection, and sclerosing agents. Traumatic sialoceles commonly arise from injury to the parotid duct. Treatment of sialoceles from acute parotid duct injury and for delayed presentations after injury are discussed. Ranulas are a subtype of mucocele from the sublingual gland classified as superficial or plunging. Treatment of ranulas must address the sublingual gland.

Transoral Sialolithotomy Without Endoscopes: An Alternative Approach to Salivary Stones   553

Janyn Quiz and M. Boyd Gillespie

 Video content accompanies this article at http://www.oto.theclinics. com.

Sialoendoscopy is a valuable technique for a variety of obstructive and nonobstructive disorders of the major salivary glands. However, the utility of sialoscopes is limited for salivary stones, which frequently required open removal. Transoral sialolithotomy without scopes is an efficient, low-cost alternative with excellent outcomes available for most of the submandibular stones.

Soft Tissue Reconstruction of Parotidectomy Defect   567

Jennifer Moy, Mark K. Wax, and Myriam Loyo

This article provides a review of soft tissue reconstructive options for the parotidectomy defect, including skin incision, primary closure, acellular dermis, autologous fat transfer, local and regional flaps, and free tissue transfer. The authors discuss considerations for volume enhancement, skin coverage, prevention of Frey syndrome, tumor surveillance, and potential complications.

Cosmetic Approaches to Parotidectomy   583

C. Alessandra Colaianni and Jeremy D. Richmon

The parotid gland is located in a cosmetically sensitive area. Given cultural emphasis on cosmesis, using minimally invasive or hidden incisions, when appropriate, can significantly improve patient satisfaction and quality of life following surgery. Facelift-style incisions have been used since the late 1960s to approach parotid pathology. Several alternative incisions, including technology-assisted approaches, also have been described in the literature. To that end, this article explores the existing data regarding several historical and emerging cosmetic approaches to the parotid gland comparing relative advantages and disadvantages of each.

Observation Rather than Surgery for Benign Parotid Tumors: Why, When, and How   593

Barak Ringel and Dennis Kraus

Surgery is the preferred treatment of benign parotid lesions, but it carries a risk of complications. Therefore, the approach toward the surgery of these lesions should seek to avoid complications. There are no guidelines or recommendations for when not to operate. Integration of comorbidities and other factors shift the scales from surgery toward observation in a small subset of patients presenting with parotid tumors. When observation is chosen, the patient should be followed frequently and cautiously, and the surgeon should be prepared to change strategy to surgical excision if in doubt.

Management Options for Sialadenosis   605

Andrew B. Davis and Henry T. Hoffman

Sialadenosis (sialosis) is a chronic, noninflammatory, nonneoplastic, bilateral, often painless enlargement of the salivary glands, most frequently affecting the parotid glands. Approximately 50% of cases are associated with an underlying disease process. The pathogenesis of sialadenosis is unknown but likely results from an autonomic neuropathy. The key to management is diagnosis and management of any poorly controlled underlying medical process.

Salivary Malignancy

Molecular Markers that Matter in Salivary Malignancy   613

Katherine C. Wai, Hyunseok Kang, and Patrick K. Ha

Despite aggressive initial interventions, recurrent/metastatic salivary gland cancer is not uncommon. Standard chemotherapy has not been shown to have durable clinical benefits. Several potential molecular markers have been identified in different histologic subtypes of salivary cancers. The objective of this review is to highlight the molecular markers that have been targeted in clinical trials for salivary gland cancers.

The Evaluation and Management of Carcinoma of the Minor Salivary Glands   629

Rohan Walvekar and Neelam Prakash Phalke

There are several hundred minor salivary glands throughout the upper aerodigestive tract, aiding in lubrication and protection of the system. Compared with all tumors of the head and neck and those of the six major glands, neoplasms of the minor glands are rare. However, more than half are found to be malignant, prompting a low threshold for further work-up. This review discusses the evaluation of patients who present with masses of the minor salivary glands, including strategies for tissue diagnosis and staging. Management options for and long-term survival outcomes of the most common malignancies affecting these glands are also discussed.

Extent and Indications for Elective and Therapeutic Neck Dissection for Salivary Carcinoma   641

Alexandra E. Kejner and Brianna N. Harris

Although salivary gland malignancies account for only a small percentage of all head and neck cancers, the incidence is increasing. Furthermore, there is a wide variety of histologic subtypes in the context of their location. Each one is associated with different rates of regional metastasis and overall survival. This article examines the incidence of salivary gland malignancies and provides evidence for the indications for and extent of elective or therapeutic neck dissection based on location, pathologic type, and histopathologic characteristics.

Special Article Series: Intentionally Shaping the Future of Otolaryngology

Foreword: Turning Dreams and Goals into Plans and Actions that Enhance
Otolaryngology   xvii

Sujana S. Chandrasekhar

Preface: From Desire to Doing   xxi

Jennifer A. Villwock

Diversifying Researchers and Funding in Otolaryngology   653

Christina H. Fang, Gregory L. Barinsky, Stacey T. Gray, Soly Baredes, Sujana S.
Chandrasekhar, and Jean Anderson Eloy

Research productivity is a key metric used in evaluation for advancement
and promotion in academic medicine. There are known gender, race, and
ethnicity disparities in otolaryngology research and funding. Female academic otolaryngologists have been shown to lag in scholarly productivity,
representation at national meetings, leadership positions on journal editorial boards, and National Institutes of Health and industry funding. Underrepresented minorities have been shown to be less successful at obtaining
Centralized Otolaryngology Research Efforts grant funding. Directed approaches, such as research funding for women and minorities or targeted
recruitment and retention of underrepresented faculty, may move the field
toward parity.

Critical Components of Diversity Initiatives   665

Brandon I. Esianor, Nicole Kloosterman, Cristina Cabrera-Muffly, David J. Brown,
and Kimberly N. Vinson

The importance of diversity is well established and holds important implications for workplace and physician-patient relationships. Evaluation of diversity statistics within otolaryngology–head and neck surgery reveals
areas of deficiency that may be improved with targeted proactive approaches. This article provides a general overview of diversity within
otolaryngology, highlights key components of diversity initiatives, and provides strategies for implementation.

OTOLARYNGOLOGIC CLINICS OF NORTH AMERICA

FORTHCOMING ISSUES

August 2021
Biologics in Otolaryngology
Sarah K. Wise, Ashkan Monfared, and
Nicole C. Schmitt, *Editors*

October 2021
The Dizzy Patient
Meredith E. Adams and Maja Svrakic,
Editors

December 2021
Childhood Hearing Loss
Nancy M. Young and Anne Marie Tharpe,
Editors

RECENT ISSUES

April 2021
Head and Neck Cutaneous Cancer
Cecelia E. Schmalbach and Kelly M.
Malloy, *Editors*

February 2021
Endoscopic Ear Surgery
Manuela X. Fina, Justin S. Golub, Daniel J.
Lee, *Editors*

December 2020
Robotics in Otolaryngology
Umamaheswar Duvvuri, Arun Sharma,
and Erica R. Thaler, *Editors*

SERIES OF RELATED INTEREST

Facial Plastic Surgery Clinics
Available at: https://www.facialplastic.theclinics.com/

THE CLINICS ARE AVAILABLE ONLINE!
Access your subscription at:
www.theclinics.com

Foreword

Salivary Gland Disease: A Comprehensive Resource

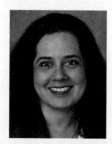

Sujana S. Chandrasekhar, MD, FACS, FAAOHNS
Consulting Editor

When I was a little girl, my mother, a pediatrician, gave us a book called *Minnie the Mump* that my sister and I read and reread over and over. That was my first under-standing of what salivary glands were, what they did, and what could go wrong with them.

Salivary glands can be viewed as the unheralded workers of major life and quality-of-life functions. We don't pay attention to their vital functions until something goes wrong. Suddenly, there's severe dry mouth or a painful (or not) swelling of the face or upper chin, or a fluid-filled lump in the mouth, and the major and minor salivary glands are front and center. Most conditions affecting salivary glands are benign, but all can be challenging to treat.

Drs Gillespie and Ryan have compiled this valuable, comprehensive, single-source issue of *Otolaryngologic Clinics of North America* that covers the most up-to-date, thorough discussion of all that one should be considering when approaching the salivary glands. The authors of these 15 articles have covered each aspect of the subject well. As surgeons, our scope of practice extends to using ultrasonography and sialoen-doscopy wisely, understanding immune-mediated pathologic conditions, as well as providing cosmetically pleasing approaches for addressing benign tumors, with facial nerve monitoring used when appropriate. Stone management has evolved, and different techniques are explained. Salivary gland malignancies are uncommon, but their management is covered, from identifying the molecular markers that matter, to treatment of the gland, and when and how to treat the neck

While Paul Tripp's book may have whet the appetite, this issue of *Otolaryngologic Clinics of North America* provides a 15-course smorgasbord of practical and enlight-ening information. The novice Otolaryngology trainee as well as the experienced

Otolaryngol Clin N Am 54 (2021) xiii–xiv
https://doi.org/10.1016/j.otc.2021.04.010
0030-6665/21/© 2021 Published by Elsevier Inc.

oto.theclinics.com

Otolaryngologic surgeon out in practice, alike, will benefit from reading all of the articles in this issue and then holding onto it as a reference in their office.

Sujana S. Chandrasekhar, MD, FACS, FAAOHNS
Consulting Editor
Otolaryngologic Clinics of North America
Past President
American Academy of Otolaryngology–
Head and Neck Surgery
Secretary-Treasurer
American Otological Society
Partner, ENT & Allergy Associates LLP
18 East 48th Street, 2nd Floor
New York, NY 10017, USA

Clinical Professor, Department of Otolaryngology–
Head and Neck Surgery
Zucker School of Medicine at Hofstra-Northwell
Hempstead, NY, USA

Clinical Associate Professor
Department of Otolaryngology–
Head and Neck Surgery
Icahn School of Medicine at Mount Sinai
New York, NY, USA

E-mail address:
ssc@nyotology.com

Website:
http://www.ears.nyc

Preface

The Science and Art of Salivary Care

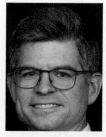 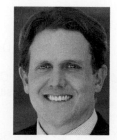

M. Boyd Gillespie, MD, MSC   William R. Ryan, MD, FACS
Editors

The salivary glands are among the body's low-profile organs that perform critical, if often overlooked functions for the organism. Salivary glands perform essential roles in oral lubrication; mastication; digestion; dental protection; articulation; and immune function. These baseline functions are often overlooked until there is a problem. When a salivary problem does occur, it is the purview of the otolaryngologist to serve as the primary problem solver. The primary challenge is that salivary diseases are common uncommon disorders. Although complaints of salivary pain and swelling are common, the frequent symptoms arise from a myriad of uncommon causes from benign and malignant tumors, inflammatory disorders, autoimmune conditions, infections, and physical obstructions. The key to successful management of salivary disorders requires the integration of science, including novel evidence and technology, with art of medical care, including diagnostic savvy and empiric interventions.

This current issue provides an up-to-date guide on perplexing salivary issues not uncommonly encountered by the otolaryngologist. The common theme that binds these articles together is the use of clinical skills, appropriate imaging, and tissue sampling to make an accurate and timely diagnosis to inform a targeted treatment plan. The issue starts with *Basics* of salivary care, including the use of in-office ultrasound to diagnose a wide range of disorders in noninvasive fashion; a review of surgical situations, which may benefit the most from facial nerve monitoring; and an overview of immunoglobulin G4–related disorders, which are difficult to diagnose but often affect the salivary glands. The section on *Surgical Techniques* focuses on patient friendly, minimally invasive approaches to the salivary gland, which preserve salivary function while minimizing morbidity. The final section on *Salivary Malignancy* provides the latest evidence regarding molecular targeted therapy for various salivary gland tumors, and new considerations in the management minor salivary cancer and regional neck disease.

Otolaryngol Clin N Am 54 (2021) xv–xvi
https://doi.org/10.1016/j.otc.2021.03.004
0030-6665/21/© 2021 Published by Elsevier Inc.

We have tried to maintain the flow of salivary gland information for our readers, who in turn must maintain the flow of these critical glands for their patients.

M. Boyd Gillespie, MD, MSC
UTHSC Otolaryngology–
Head and Neck Surgery
University of Tennessee Health Science Center
910 Madison Avenue, Suite 408
Memphis, TN 38163, USA

William R. Ryan, MD, FACS
Department of Otolaryngology–
Head and Neck Surgery
Helen Diller Comprehensive Cancer Center
University of California, San Francisco
Mission Bay Medical Center
1825 4th Street, 5th Floor
San Francisco, CA 94158, USA

E-mail addresses:
mgilles8@uthsc.edu (M.B. Gillespie)
William.Ryan@ucsf.edu (W.R. Ryan)

BASICS

Practical Salivary Ultrasound Imaging Tips and Pearls

Mary Jue Xu, MD, Jolie L. Chang, MD*

KEYWORDS

- Ultrasound imaging • Salivary gland • Clinical exam • Salivary pathology

KEY POINTS

- Familiarity with normal salivary gland anatomy and proper probe placement is essential for ultrasound salivary gland examinations.
- Characteristic ultrasound findings for sialolithiasis, salivary duct stenosis, neoplasms, and autoimmune salivary disorders are demonstrated.
- The anterior floor of mouth is difficult to visualize on ultrasound; bimanual examination with intraoral palpation and transcervical probe placement enhances visualization of pathology in this area.
- Ultrasound guidance augments fine-needle aspiration biopsies of lesions, salivary gland injections, and sialendoscopic-assisted surgeries.

INTRODUCTION

Ultrasound (US) technology has evolved into an indispensable point-of-care technology due to its ability to enhance the clinical evaluation of head and neck disorders. Its portability and low cost has propelled and redefined ultrasound utility in clinical settings globally.[1,2]

In US probes, piezoelectric crystals convert between mechanical energy and electricity. Electric charges delivered deform these crystals and generate high-frequency sound waves that are dispersed into tissue. These sound waves deflect off of tissue with a portion returning back to the probe. Sound waves returning to the probe are then converted to electric energy and transformed into an image on the ultrasound monitor. The most commonly used probes for head and neck imaging are 7 to 15 MHz high-frequency linear array transducers. Higher-frequency transducers allow for better image resolution but are compromised by lower tissue penetration

Department of Otolaryngology–Head and Neck Surgery, University of California San Francisco, 2380 Sutter Street Box 0342, San Francisco, CA 94115, USA
* Corresponding author.
E-mail address: jolie.chang@ucsf.edu

Otolaryngol Clin N Am 54 (2021) 471–487
https://doi.org/10.1016/j.otc.2021.02.008
0030-6665/21/Published by Elsevier Inc.
oto.theclinics.com

The major advantages of ultrasonography are the capabilities for immediate dynamic imaging, intraoperative use, and avoidance of radiation. Unlike computed tomography (CT) imaging, lack of radiation makes this technology safe for repeat examinations in children and pregnant patients. US also offers real-time, dynamic, and targeted 2-dimensional imaging. Similar to all imaging modalities (**Table 1**), US imaging has limitations including operator dependency and incomplete visualization of deep and obstructed structures.

SALIVARY GLAND ANATOMY

On US, normal salivary gland parenchyma is homogeneous and hyperechoic compared with surrounding tissues due to the higher fat content of the glands. As the probe is moved, vessels are followed longitudinally in comparison with focal lymph nodes or salivary gland lesions that appear and disappear from view as the probe moves. Motion of the probe is essential for delineating and defining structures.

Parotid Gland

The deep and superficial lobes of the parotid gland are delineated by the facial nerve intraoperatively and retromandibular vein radiologically. The facial nerve and its branches cannot be directly visualized on US. However, the retromandibular vein marks the relative depth of the facial nerve.[3] Lesion location can be defined relative to this landmark. Accessory parotid glands are found in 20% of patients adjacent to the main parotid duct and projecting superficial to the masseter muscle.[4]

The main parotid duct exits the hilum of the gland and courses superficial to the masseter muscle approximately 1 cm inferior to the zygomatic arch before piercing the buccinator muscle and entering the oral cavity opposite the second maxillary molar. Normal ducts cannot routinely be visualized on US. Dilated ducts are seen as an anechoic tract on US running from the parotid hilum and superficial to the masseter muscle. Dilated ducts are a sign of duct obstruction most often caused by stones or duct stenosis. If a dilated duct is visualized, it can be followed to the "pinch point" of obstruction distally.

Submandibular Gland

The submandibular gland sits medially in the upper neck. Laterally, it is adjacent to the tail of the parotid gland. Medially, it wraps around the posterior edge of the mylohyoid muscle, which is called the uncinate process. The submandibular duct, or Wharton's duct, exits the submandibular gland hilum and travels around the dorsal edge of the mylohyoid muscle into the floor of mouth. The duct then traverses through the sublingual gland to the papilla in the anterior floor of mouth.

Sublingual Gland

The sublingual gland is situated within the floor of mouth superior to the mylohyoid muscle between the mandible and tongue. The submandibular duct runs along the medial aspect of the sublingual gland.[5]

ULTRASOUND TECHNIQUE
Setup and Approach

Patients should be seated and comfortable. To elongate the neck, the patient is reclined and the chin is turned to the opposite side of the area being examined. Ensure proper probe orientation to the image on the screen. Examine bilateral major salivary glands in a systematic manner and focus on gland size and texture, presence of

Table 1
Comparison of salivary gland imaging modalities

Imaging Modality	Ultrasound	Computed Tomography	MRI	Sialography
Advantages	• Real-time, point-of-care diagnosis • Cost-effective • No radiation • No contrast required • Allows for real-time procedure guidance	• Good for evaluating calcifications, bony erosion • Used in acute settings: abscesses or deep neck space infections	• Characterization of salivary gland masses given excellent soft tissue contrast and resolution • Evaluates perineural invasion, tumor margins, deep space involvement such as parapharyngeal space • No radiation	• Assessment of the entire duct anatomy including all branches
Disadvantages	• Operator dependent • Limited evaluation depth	• Radiation exposure • May require contrast for visualization • Separate appointment required	• Patient tolerance/claustrophobia • Time • Cost • Limited by metallic implants, pacemakers • Separate appointment required	• Requires expertise to cannulate the duct for contrast infusion in the duct • Radiation exposure

lesions, and visibility of the duct. One approach to a systematic examination is presented as follows (**Fig. 1**).

Submandibular and Sublingual Glands
1. Lateral transverse view (see **Fig. 1**A, B)
   - Place the probe in a transverse orientation along the inferior border of the mandible.
   - Scan between mandible and the level of the hyoid bone to assess the full extent of the submandibular gland. Visualize the submandibular gland hilum at the posterior border of the mylohyoid muscle and follow the trajectory of the submandibular duct toward the sublingual gland deep to the mylohyoid.
   - Use bimanual palpation of the floor of the mouth to enhance visualization of lesions along the duct trajectory by pushing the floor of mouth tissue with a gloved finger against the US transducer that is placed on the neck.
   - To visualize the sublingual gland, move the probe parallel to the mandible body and angle the probe superiorly. The sublingual gland is deep to the mylohyoid on the image.
2. Midline transverse view (see **Fig. 1**C, D)
   - Place the probe in an axial orientation at the midline submental space.
   - Assess tissues within level 1a of the neck by scanning between the symphysis and hyoid.
   - The mylohyoid muscle can be more closely examined laterally. For plunging ranulas of the sublingual gland, which will appear as an anechoic mass, the location where the ranula pierces the mylohyoid can be evaluated.

Parotid Gland
1. Transverse view of the parotid tail (see **Fig. 1**E, F)
   - Place the probe in a transverse position inferior to the ear lobule.
   - Scan infra-auricularly to examine the parotid tail. A portion of the deep lobe of the parotid is seen between the mastoid and mandible. In this view, the retromandibular vein estimates the depth of the facial nerve.
2. Longitudinal pre-auricular view (see **Fig. 1**G, H)
   - Place the probe vertically anterior to the tragus with the marker pointing cephalad.
   - Visualize the main body of the gland posterior to the masseter muscle and inferiorly the parotid tail adjacent to the sternocleidomastoid muscle.
3. Anterior transverse view (see **Fig. 1**I, J)
   - Place the probe in the transverse orientation across the cheek between the tragus and the oral commissure.
   - Visualize the course of the parotid duct. The main parotid duct traverses through the gland hilum and over the masseter muscle, approximately 1 cm inferior to the zygomatic arch.
   - Assess for accessory parotid duct, which can be found in 20% of patients adjacent to the parotid duct and projecting over the masseter.

Lymph nodes
For workup of neoplasms, assess the surrounding lymph nodes in all levels of the neck. Normal lymph nodes have a hyperechoic linear hilum, have hilar pattern blood flow on Doppler, and are often ovoid in shape. Malignant lymph nodes are rounded, larger than 1 cm, have absent hilum, have more erratic or generalized blood flow on Doppler, and may contain microcalcifications, cysts, or internal necrosis (**Fig. 2**). In addition to augmenting the clinical examination, ultrasound may also be used for US-guided fine-needle aspiration

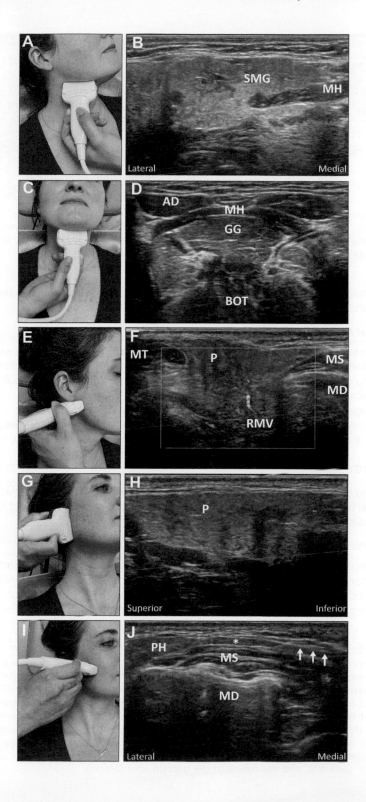

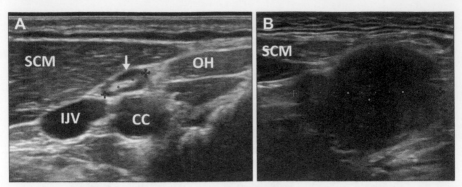

Fig. 2. Transverse view of the right neck with adjacent sternocleidomastoid (SCM), omo-hyoid (OH), internal jugular vein (IJV), and common carotid (CC) (*A*). A normal lymph node (*arrow*) has a fatty hyperechoic hilum with vascular flow on Doppler. A malignant lymph node can have irregular, ill-defined borders without visible hilum (*B*).

(FNA), which has increased sensitivity, specificity, and accuracy than FNA without US.[6]

Additional Maneuvers

Bimanual sono-palpation is performed with digital palpation intraorally and the US probe externally on the neck or face. The gloved finger is directed either at the buccal mucosa to define lesions near the parotid duct papilla or at the floor of mouth for the submandibular and sublingual gland pathologies (**Fig. 3**).

Sialagogues stimulate saliva generation and can enhance visualization of dilated salivary ducts during examination. Sialagogues include lemon candies, lemon wedges, or citric acid crystals.

PATHOLOGY

In allowing clinicians to augment their clinical examination, ultrasound enhances the evaluation for salivary gland pathologies including sialadenitis, salivary duct stenosis, sialolithiasis, autoimmune-related diseases, and tumors.

Sialadenitis

Sialadenitis, or salivary gland inflammation, has a broad differential.[7] Acute inflammation is often viral or bacterial in origin. Causes of chronic inflammation include pro-longed duct obstruction from internal (ie, sialolithiasis, duct stenosis) or external pathologies (ie, tumor compression). Additional causes of sialadenitis include

Fig. 1. Approach to US examination of the salivary glands. (*A, B*) Lateral transverse view of the right submandibular gland (SMG) wrapping around the mylohyoid muscle (MH). (*C, D*) Midline, transverse view. The bilateral anterior digastric muscles (AG) are seen next to the mylohyoid and genioglossus muscles (GG). BOT, base of tongue. (*E, F*) Transverse view of the tail of the parotid (P) is between the mastoid bone (MT), masseter muscle (MS), and mandible (MD). The location of the retromandibular vein (RMV) with Doppler flow approx-imates the depth of the facial nerve. (*G, H*) Longitudinal, pre-auricular view of the parotid. (*I, J*) Anterior, transverse view of the parotid highlights the parotid hilum (PH), accessory pa-rotid tissue (*asterisk*), and the course of the parotid duct (*arrow*).

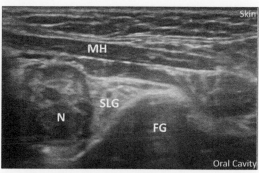

Fig. 3. Bimanual palpation during US helps localize and identify lesions. The nodule (N) in the left floor of mouth is best visualized in the sublingual gland (SLG) with assistance of a gloved intraoral finger (FG). MH, mylohyoid.

autoimmune or immune-mediated diseases, radioactive iodine therapy, and salivary gland tumors.

Compared with normal homogeneous salivary glands, acutely infected glands are diffusely enlarged, heterogeneous with hypoechoic regions, and have increased vascular flow (**Fig. 4**). Glands should be assessed for sialoliths that may be causing obstruction.

Chronically obstructed glands can become atrophied (**Fig. 5**). On US, glands appear shrunken, isoechoic, and heterogeneous with little recognizable parenchyma. Salivary gland atrophy can also result from radiotherapy, radioactive iodine, autoimmune diseases, chronic ductal obstruction, or other causes of chronic sialadenitis.[8]

Sialolithiasis

Sialolithiasis is most common in the submandibular gland (60%–80% of cases) in comparison with the parotid gland (6%–15%) and sublingual and minor salivary glands (2%).[9,10]

On US, stones appear as hyperechoic curvilinear lines with posterior/deep acoustic shadowing (**Fig. 6**). US examination can diagnose and localize the stone. US has an 84% sensitivity and 100% specificity for detecting salivary calculi larger than 2 mm, with smaller stones lacking the posterior/deep shadowing and being more challenging to palpate.[11] Stones in the anterior floor of mouth are particularly challenging to visualize on US; thus, such stones may require bimanual sonopalpation.

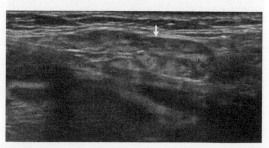

Fig. 4. Acute sialadenitis of the left submandibular gland is marked by diffuse hypoechoic changes within the parenchyma (*arrow*).

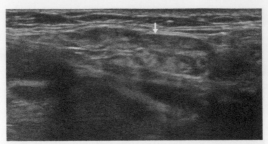

Fig. 5. Left submandibular gland atrophy (*arrow*) with chronic sialadenitis is characterized by a smaller gland with heterogeneous echotexture.

Imaging localization of sialoliths can inform surgical approach, particularly in the case of parotid sialoliths. Sialoliths in the proximal parotid duct posterior to the masseter may require a combined sialendoscopic transfacial approach in contrast to sialoliths in the distal duct near the papilla that can often be managed with transoral approaches.[12]

Stenosis or Stricture

Ductal obstruction from salivary duct stones and duct stenoses can result in ductal dilation proximal to the obstruction. A dilated duct appears anechoic and tubelike. In contrast to blood vessels, dilated ducts do not show internal blood flow on Doppler (**Fig. 7**). US can help identify the course of the duct and assist with duct instrumentation for treatment with sialendoscopy. Preoperative knowledge of the stricture or stenosis location assists with surgical planning and discussion of outcomes. Larson et al.[13] reported that patients with distal duct (closer to papilla) stenosis had greater symptomatic relief following sialendoscopy compared with patients with more proximal stenoses (intraglandular).

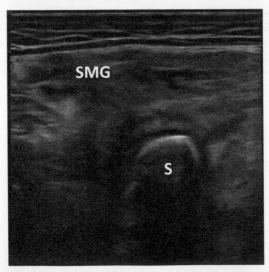

Fig. 6. Sialolithiasis (S) of the left submandibular gland (SMG) appears as a curvilinear, hyperechoic line with posterior acoustic shadowing.

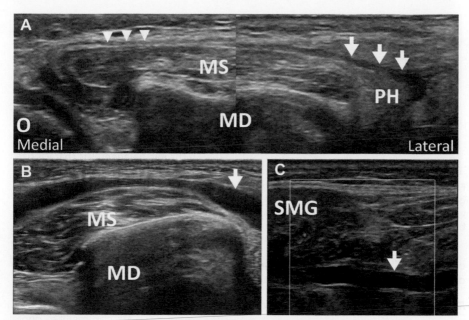

Fig. 7. Salivary ducts appear as anechoic, dilated tubular structures. Left proximal dilated parotid duct (*A, arrows*) is seen within the parotid hilum (PH); the main duct over the masseter muscle is normal caliber (*arrowhead*), suggesting a proximal duct stenosis. Megaduct (*arrow*) is an example of distal parotid duct stenosis with severe main duct dilation (*B*). (*C*) Right submandibular duct dilation (*arrow*) is suggestive of distal duct obstruction. MD, mandible; MS, masseter muscle; O, oral cavity; SMG, submandibular gland.

Sjogren's Syndrome

Although diagnostic criteria proposed by the American-European Consensus Group propose specific findings for Sjogren's syndrome diagnosis include xerostomia, salivary gland swelling, and abnormal Schirmer test,[14] there is growing recognition and validation of US findings as valuable for diagnosing Sjogren's syndrome.[15] On US, parotid glands with Sjogren's syndrome appear heterogeneous with hypoechoic regions; these findings represent dilated ducts and enlarged lymph nodes, suggestive of degenerative and inflammatory parenchymal damage[5] (**Fig. 8**). Multiple glands are typically affected. Submandibular glands are often heterogeneous and atrophic on US. Multiple intraparenchymal calcifications, which do not represent intraductal stones, can be found in some patients, suggesting immune-mediated disease.[16]

Immunoglobulin G4-Related Diseases of the Salivary Gland

Immunoglobulin (Ig)G4-related diseases are marked by dense infiltration of predominantly IgG4-positive plasma cells in tissues and vessels around the body often accompanied with fibrotic changes and increased eosinophils.[17] Patients with IgG4-related sialadenitis often have associated allergic rhinitis, bronchial asthma, and autoimmune pancreatitis, and less often xerostomia and dry eyes.[18] Mikulicz disease, Kuttner tumor (sclerosing sialadenitis), and Riedel thyroiditis are all now grouped under IgG4-related diseases.[19]

Clinically, affected salivary glands can be firm and significantly enlarged. On US, findings demonstrate diffuse salivary gland enlargement with heterogeneous

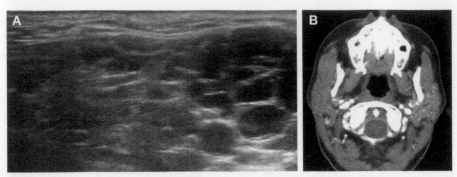

Fig. 8. Sjogren's syndrome is characterized by heterogeneous, multicystic, hypoechoic regions that represent dilated ducts and enlarged lymph nodes (A, right parotid sagittal view). On CT imaging, intraparenchymal calcifications in the bilateral parotid glands can be seen (B).

echotexture[20] (**Fig. 9**). Blood IgG4 levels are elevated in two-thirds of patients.[21] The disease responds well to corticosteroids.

Radioactive Iodine-Induced Sialadenitis

Following administration of radioactive iodine (RAI), up to 40% of patients demonstrate salivary obstruction or xerostomia symptoms in the first year following RAI and 5% with persistent symptoms at 7 years.[22] In a study of 202 patients, post-RAI gland changes were found in 46.5% (94) of patients on US examinations 1 to 2 years after RAI therapy.[23]

US findings are similar to chronic sialadenitis and include changes in echogenicity and gland atrophy indicative of gland degeneration. Echotexture changes related to RAI are more commonly seen in the parotid gland (46.0%) compared with the submandibular gland (3.5%).[23]

Human Immunodeficiency Virus Parotid Lymphoepithelial Cysts

Benign parotid lymphoepithelial cysts occur in 3% to 6% of patients infected with human immunodeficiency virus (HIV). The cysts are thought to occur from secondary gland and duct obstruction due to intraparotid lymph node hyperplasia.[24] On imaging, lesions appear as mixed cystic and solid lesions in the parotid gland with associated gland enlargement and cervical lymphadenopathy (**Fig. 10**).

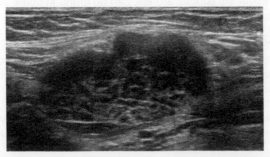

Fig. 9. IgG4-related salivary gland disease presents as diffusely enlarged glands with heterogeneous echotexture.

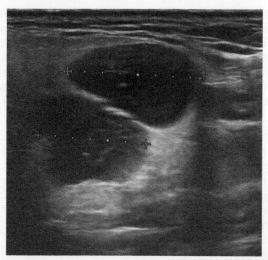

Fig. 10. HIV-related lymphoepithelial cysts appear as hypoechoic cysts in the parotid parenchyma, seen on sagittal view of the right inferior parotid tail. Biopsy of these lesions noted follicular hyperplasia.

Neoplasms

Neoplasms of the salivary glands include both benign pathologies such as pleomorphic adenoma and Warthin tumor, as well as malignant lesions (**Fig. 11**). On US, lesion characteristics including the mass size, shape, borders, vascularity, content, and adjacent lymph nodes should all be noted. Pleomorphic adenomas are often hypoechoic, lobulated lesions with well-defined borders and deep enhancement, and

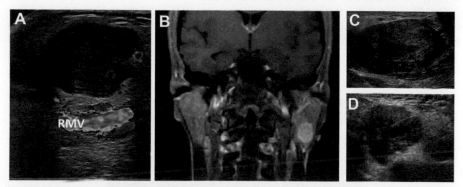

Fig. 11. Benign and malignant salivary gland lesions cannot be clearly distinguished; lesions require FNA biopsy for diagnosis. Pleomorphic adenomas appear as well-circumscribed, multilobulated, hypoechoic lesions seen on US (*A*) and on T1-weighted MRI with contrast (*B*). Warthin tumors are heterogeneous and hypoechoic with anechoic cystic regions and internal vascularity (*C*). Metastatic cutaneous squamous cell carcinoma appears as a hypoechoic lesion with cystic changes and poorly defined borders (*D*). RMV, retromandibular vein.

sometimes contain hyperechoic elements suggestive of calcifications. Warthin tumors are hypoechoic, well-defined lesions that can contain anechoic cystic regions, are often hypervascular, and can appear bilaterally.[25] In contrast to benign lesions, malignant lesions can appear hypoechoic, heterogeneous, and hypervascular and have irregular shapes and infiltrative borders. The distinction between benign and malignant lesions on ultrasound is often not apparent. FNA biopsy is required for additional diagnostic information.[26]

Benign Masseteric Hypertrophy

Masseter muscle hypertrophy can be confused with salivary gland hypertrophy and disease. Patients may present with facial swelling along the mandibular body and or mid-cheek. Examination findings of masseter muscle pain and history of bruxism supplement the diagnosis. US imaging at the location of fullness demonstrates an enlarged masseter muscle (**Fig. 12**). Significant masseteric hypertrophy can laterally displace and narrow the Stenson duct.[27]

Vascular Malformation

Vascular malformations are the most common congenital vascular lesion of the salivary glands, but can occur at any age in the setting of hormone changes, trauma, or infection.[28] In some cases, blood stasis can lead to formation of phleboliths, or calcified blood clots, which can be confused with sialoliths. On US, phleboliths appear as hyperechoic lesions adjacent to or within the salivary gland tissue.[29] Demonstration of increased internal vascularity on US with Doppler can aid with vascular malformation evaluation; however, multiplanar imaging with contrast are often necessary to confirm the diagnosis.

Ranula

Obstructed sublingual glands can lead to the formation of a ranula. These are pseudocysts without an epithelial lining. Ranulas are classified as either simple when contained in the sublingual space, or plunging, when extending inferior to the mylohyoid muscle into the submandibular space.

On US, ranulas are thin-walled, anechoic cysts with loculations (**Fig. 13**). Infection can lead to a more echogenic appearance. For plunging ranulas, US can be used to find the site where the ranula traverses the mylohyoid and attaches to the sublingual

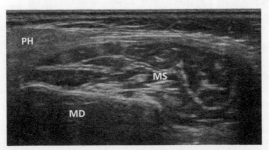

Fig. 12. Benign masseteric hypertrophy on US is noted for normal-appearing salivary glands with facial fullness corresponding to an enlarged masseter muscle (MS). MD, mandible; PH, parotid hilum.

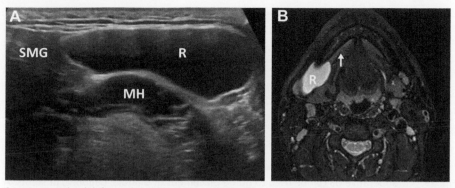

Fig. 13. Ranulas (R) from the sublingual gland, appear as thin-walled, anechoic masses that may contain loculations. Ranula (R) collection is seen anterior to the right submandibular gland (SMG) (*A*). On MRI T2 sequence (*B*), the cystic portion of this plunging ranula extends to the sublingual gland (*arrow*). MH, mylohyoid.

gland. Management with transoral resection of sublingual gland and ranula cavity decompression is associated with the lowest rates of recurrence.[30]

PROCEDURES
Fine-Needle Aspiration Biopsy

US guidance can localize lesions for biopsy and aspiration. The location and depth of the lesion determines the appropriate needle placement and trajectory relative to the US probe. With the lesion visualized, the operator's dominant hand directs the needle underneath the probe. The relationship between the US probe and needle can be either perpendicular (short axis) or parallel (long axis, **Fig. 14**). Choice of approach

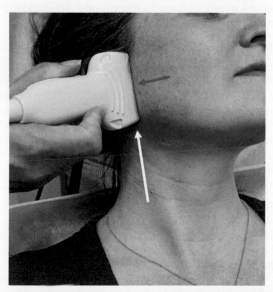

Fig. 14. US-guided needle placement for biopsy or injection. Needle-directed localization can be performed in either short-axis (*short blue arrow*) or the long-axis (*long white arrow*) trajectories in relation to the US probe. Furthermore, these approaches can be combined if needed.

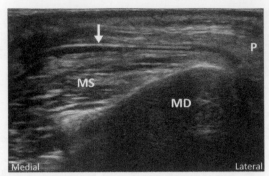

Fig. 15. Intraoperative US can be used to guide placement of dilators, balloons, or stents. A stent was placed in the main left parotid duct (*arrow*). MD, mandible; MS, masseter muscle; P, parotid.

depends on the position and depth of the target. The long-axis approach allows for visualization of the entire needle trajectory into the lesion; thus, this approach is often preferred.

ULTRASOUND-GUIDED BOTULINUM TOXIN INJECTION

Botulinum toxin injections are used for treating sialorrhea, chronic sialadenitis, sialoceles, and salivary fistulas. Protocols vary in the number of units to use for each gland depending on the purpose and diagnosis.[31] For persistent chronic sialadenitis, sialocele, or salivary fistula, 60 to 100 units of onabotulinum toxin A equivalent can be injected into the gland. For sialorrhea, 100 units or more are often distributed between the 4 major salivary glands. The exact amount can be individualized based on response. US guidance allows delivery to the salivary gland parenchyma and avoidance of blood vessels and muscles.

Ultrasound Guidance in Conjunction with Sialendoscopy and Surgical Interventions

US can supplement surgical approaches in the operating room and should be used to confirm pathology of interest. In the case of sialolithiasis, US provides confirmation of stone location and number before sialendoscopic surgery. After removal, US helps identify any remaining sialoliths and confirms complete removal. Furthermore, intraoperative US localization of proximal parotid stones assists with minimally invasive transparotidotomy approaches for stone removal. US also can assist in salivary duct dilation and instrumentation (**Fig. 15**). In complex cases, US needle guidance helps access the main duct and assist with duct repair.[32]

SUMMARY

US is an indispensable point-of-care technology that enhances clinical examination and evaluation of head and neck pathology. Notable and distinctive salivary gland findings include acute or chronic sialadenitis with enlarged and heterogeneous glands, sialolithiasis with hyperechoic curvilinear structures with posterior/deep acoustic shadowing, and autoimmune diseases such as Sjogren's syndrome with heterogeneous multicystic gland degeneration with multiple hypoechoic regions. US guidance can enhance needle localization for procedures such as FNA biopsies and gland injections. Intraoperative ultrasound can enhance surgical identification of sialoliths and strictures to better enable surgical therapies.

CLINICS CARE POINTS

- For sialolithiasis, US examination shows a hyperechoic rim with posterior shadowing. Understanding sialolith location, size, and number assists with surgical planning.
- The anterior floor of mouth is difficult to visualize on US; bimanual examination enhances visualization of pathology in this area.
- US visualization of dilated salivary ducts suggests obstructive pathology distal (closer to papilla) to the dilation. Duct stenosis location and size assists with surgical planning and outcomes.
- Sjogren's syndrome appears with distinctive heterogeneous parenchyma with multiple hypoechoic regions within both parotid glands.
- Salivary gland neoplasms may require FNA biopsy given the challenges in distinguishing benign from malignant lesions based on US features alone.
- US can aid the diagnosis of masseter muscle hypertrophy, vascular malformations, and ranulas.
- US guidance assists with FNA biopsies and salivary gland injections.
- Intraoperative US provides real-time evaluation and localization of sialoliths and strictures to better enable surgical therapy.

DISCLOSURE

J.L. Chang and M.J. Xu declare no conflicts of interest.

REFERENCES

1. D'Cruz AK, Vaish R, Kapre N, et al. Elective versus therapeutic neck dissection in node-negative oral cancer. N Engl J Med 2015;373(6):521–9.
2. Stewart KA, Navarro SM, Kambala S, et al. Trends in ultrasound use in low and middle income countries: a systematic review. Int J MCH AIDS 2020;9(1):103–20.
3. Jecker P, Orloff LA. Salivary gland ultrasonography. In: Orloff LA, editor. Head and neck ultrasonography. San Diego (CA): Plural Publishing; 2008. p. 129–52.
4. Harnsberger HR, Glastonbury CM. Parotid space. In: Harnsberger HR, editor. Diagnostic imaging: head and neck. Philadelphia: Amirsys; 2004. p. 2–36.
5. Bialek EJ, Jakubowski W, Zajkowski P, et al. US of the major salivary glands: anatomy and spatial relationships, pathologic conditions, and pitfalls. Radiographics 2006;26(3):745–63.
6. Baatenburg de Jong RJ, Rongen RJ, Verwoerd CD, et al. Ultrasound-guided fine-needle aspiration biopsy of neck nodes. Arch Otolaryngol Head Neck Surg 1991; 117(4):402–4.
7. Abdel Razek AAK, Mukherji S. Imaging of sialadenitis. Neuroradiol J 2017;30(3): 205–15.
8. Vissink A, Jansma J, Spijkervet FK, et al. Oral sequelae of head and neck radiotherapy. Crit Rev Oral Biol Med 2003;14(3):199–212.
9. Marchal F, Dulguerov P. Sialolithiasis management: the state of the art. Arch Otolaryngol Head Neck Surg 2003;129(9):951–6.

10. Moghe S, Pillai A, Thomas S, et al. Parotid sialolithiasis. BMJ Case Rep 2012; 2012. bcr2012007480.
11. Gritzmann N, Rettenbacher T, Hollerweger A, et al. Sonography of the salivary glands. Eur Radiol 2003;13(5):964–75.
12. Kiringoda R, Eisele DW, Chang JL. A comparison of parotid imaging characteristics and sialendoscopic findings in obstructive salivary disorders. Laryngoscope 2014;124(12):2696–701.
13. Larson AR, Aubin-Pouliot A, Delagnes E, et al. Surgeon-performed ultrasound for chronic obstructive sialadenitis helps predict sialendoscopic findings and outcomes. Otolaryngol Head Neck Surg 2017;157(6):973–80.
14. Vitali C, Bombardieri S, Jonsson R, et al. Classification criteria for Sjogren's syndrome: a revised version of the European criteria proposed by the American-European Consensus Group. Ann Rheum Dis 2002;61(6):554–8.
15. van Nimwegen JF, Mossel E, Delli K, et al. Incorporation of salivary gland ultrasonography into the American College of Rheumatology/European League Against Rheumatism criteria for primary Sjogren's Syndrome. Arthritis Care Res (Hoboken) 2020;72(4):583–90.
16. Jauregui E, Kiringoda R, Ryan WR, et al. Chronic parotitis with multiple calcifications: clinical and sialendoscopic findings. Laryngoscope 2017;127(7):1565–70.
17. Deshpande V, Zen Y, Chan JK, et al. Consensus statement on the pathology of IgG4-related disease. Mod Pathol 2012;25(9):1181–92.
18. Masaki Y, Sugai S, Umehara H. IgG4-related diseases including Mikulicz's disease and sclerosing pancreatitis: diagnostic insights. J Rheumatol 2010;37(7): 1380–5.
19. Geyer JT, Deshpande V. IgG4-associated sialadenitis. Curr Opin Rheumatol 2011;23(1):95–101.
20. Wang ZJ, Zheng LY, Pu YP, et al. Clinical features and treatment outcomes of immunoglobulin G4-related sclerosing sialadenitis. J Craniofac Surg 2014; 25(6):2089–93.
21. Carruthers MN, Khosroshahi A, Augustin T, et al. The diagnostic utility of serum IgG4 concentrations in IgG4-related disease. Ann Rheum Dis 2015;74(1):14–8.
22. Grewal RK, Larson SM, Pentlow CE, et al. Salivary gland side effects commonly develop several weeks after initial radioactive iodine ablation. J Nucl Med 2009; 50(10):1605–10.
23. Kim DW. Ultrasonographic features of the major salivary glands after radioactive iodine ablation in patients with papillary thyroid carcinoma. Ultrasound Med Biol 2015;41(10):2640–5.
24. Sujatha D, Babitha K, Prasad RS, et al. Parotid lymphoepithelial cysts in human immunodeficiency virus: a review. J Laryngol Otol 2013;127(11):1046–9.
25. Peter Klussmann J, Wittekindt C, Florian Preuss S, et al. High risk for bilateral Warthin tumor in heavy smokers–review of 185 cases. Acta Otolaryngol 2006;126(11): 1213–7.
26. Haidar YM, Moshtaghi O, Mahmoodi A, et al. The utility of in-office ultrasound in the diagnosis of parotid lesions. Otolaryngol Head Neck Surg 2017;156(3):511–7.
27. Gadodia A, Bhalla AS, Sharma R, et al. Bilateral parotid swelling: a radiological review. Dentomaxillofac Radiol 2011;40(7):403–14.
28. Ho C, Judson BL, Prasad ML. Vascular malformation with phleboliths involving the parotid gland: a case report with a review of the literature. Ear Nose Throat J 2015;94(10–11):E1–5.
29. Gooi Z, Mydlarz WK, Tunkel DE, et al. Submandibular venous malformation phleboliths mimicking sialolithiasis in children. Laryngoscope 2014;124(12):2826–8.

30. Harrison JD. Modern management and pathophysiology of ranula: literature review. Head Neck 2010;32(10):1310–20.
31. Barbero P, Busso M, Artusi CA, et al. Ultrasound-guided botulinum toxin-A injections: a method of treating sialorrhea. J Vis Exp 2016;117.
32. Ryan WR, Chang JL, Eisele DW. Surgeon-performed ultrasound and transfacial sialoendoscopy for complete parotid duct stenosis. Laryngoscope 2014;124(2): 418–20.

Indications for Facial Nerve Monitoring During Parotidectomy

Mirabelle Sajisevi, MD

KEYWORDS

- Electromyography • Facial nerve monitoring • Parotidectomy

KEY POINTS

- The facial nerve is at risk during parotid surgery due to its course through the gland and variable anatomic branching.
- Intraoperative electromyographic nerve monitoring can be used in parotid surgery to identify the facial nerve, map its course, identify surgical maneuvers that are possibly detrimental to the nerve, and provide prognostic information.
- Incidence of temporary weakness is significantly reduced with intraoperative nerve monitoring compared with unmonitored patients in primary parotidectomy.
- Permanent facial nerve paralysis has not been shown to be significantly affected by the use of nerve monitoring.

INTRODUCTION

The overall incidence of salivary gland neoplasms in the United States is 5.5 cases per 100,000 individuals for which the current first-line treatment of these tumors, whether benign or malignant, is surgical removal.[1] The facial nerve is at risk during parotid surgery due to its course through the gland delineating the deep and superficial lobes, as well as its variable anatomic branching to innervate the muscles of facial expression. Transient facial nerve dysfunction can occur in up to 65% of patients, whereas permanent injury can be seen in 6% to 9% of patients.[2,3] Depending on the degree and site of injury, facial nerve insult can range from mild weakness in one distribution of the nerve to full facial paralysis, which can significantly affect quality of life. Intraoperative facial nerve monitoring has been described as a potential means to reduce injury and morbidity from parotidectomy. This article reviews the indications for its use.

Department of Surgery, Division of Otolaryngology, University of Vermont Medical Center, 111 Colchester Avenue, Burlington, VT 05401, USA
E-mail address: Mirabelle.sajisevi@uvmhealtth.org

Otolaryngol Clin N Am 54 (2021) 489–496
https://doi.org/10.1016/j.otc.2021.02.001
0030-6665/21/© 2021 Elsevier Inc. All rights reserved.

oto.theclinics.com

HISTORY

The first example of facial nerve monitoring was reported by Krause in 1898, at which time electrical stimulation was described with visual confirmation of the response.[4] During a cochlear nerve section, he noted that "...unipolar faradaic irritation of the nerve trunk with the weakest possible current of the induction apparatus resulted in contractions of the right facial region, especially of the orbicularis oculi, as well as the branches supplying the nose and mouth...".[5] In the 1960s, dedicated facial nerve monitoring systems were designed for use during parotid and otologic surgeries.[4] Further developments in facial nerve monitoring occurred in the 1970s and 1980s. In 1979, Delgado and colleagues first described intraoperative electromyographic (EMG) facial nerve monitoring in cerebellopontine angle surgery.[4–6] Subsequent advancements included combining acoustic feedback with EMG and correlating specific patterns of activity to surgical manipulations.[4] In 1984, the "Nerve Integrity Monitor" (NIM) was developed by Kartush and Prass with Nicolet Company (Madison, WI, USA). This system was subsequently purchased by Xomed (Medtronic) whose version is now the most commonly used device in the United States.[4]

DEFINITIONS
Types of Nerve Monitoring

- Direct visualization: direct visualization of facial muscle movement with stimulation of the facial nerve. This type of mechanical monitoring requires a large suprathreshold response to observe contractions.
  - Setup: the patient is positioned and prepped for parotid surgery. A clear drape is placed in a sterile fashion over the face to allow for visualization during surgery. Typically, an assistant is then able to monitor for facial contractions to notify the surgeon when they occur.
- EMG: EMG records the electrical potentials that are generated by muscle fibers during depolarization termed "compound muscle action potentials". This is in contrast to compound nerve action potentials (CNAPs), which is the electrical activity generated by the nerve itself. Because of the natural amplifying effect of the muscle response, using the CMAP allows for an order of magnitude larger response to be observed compared with the CNAP.[7] The remainder of this article refers specifically to intraoperative EMG nerve monitoring during parotid surgery.
  - Setup: there are many systems commercially available. The NIM, as the most commonly used system in the United States, will be depicted here for demonstration. Once the patient has been properly positioned for parotid surgery, nerve electrodes are inserted into frontalis, orbicularis oculi, orbicularis oris and depressor anguli oris and secured with adhesive tape (**Fig. 1**A). Ground electrodes for the intramuscular electrodes and for the nerve stimulator are placed into the deltoid region. The electrode wires are connected to a circuit box that directly interfaces with a monitor (**Fig. 1**B). Once the patient is prepped and draped, a sterile stimulation probe is connected to the circuit box for use during surgery. Stimulation of the nerve (**Fig. 1**C) generates an auditory and visual response on the monitor (**Fig. 1**D). Typical parameters used at our institution are stimulus intensity of 0.8 mA with event threshold of 100 µV; however, preferences vary for these settings. It is important to communicate with the anesthesia team so that patients do not receive long-acting muscle relaxation, as this will interfere with muscle contraction and neural monitoring.

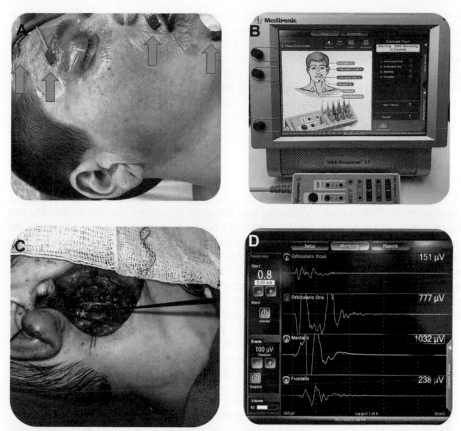

Fig. 1. Intraoperative facial nerve monitoring. (*A*) Placement of electrodes. (*B*) Circuit box and monitor. (*C*) Nerve stimulation of facial nerve trunk. (*D*) Visual response on monitor in response to facial nerve stimulation.

Types of Parotidectomy

- Extracapsular dissection: partial parotid surgery that involves removal of a tumor without exposure of the main trunk of the facial nerve.[8]
- Partial superficial parotidectomy: any procedure in which less than a superficial lobectomy is performed with only a portion of the facial nerve dissected (ie, the peripheral branches beyond the tumor site are not exposed). Stensen duct is usually preserved unless it hinders resection of the tumor.[9]
- Superficial parotidectomy: superficial lobe completely resected, involving more dissection of the facial nerve than partial superficial parotidectomy. Stenson duct is typically ligated as part of the procedure.[9]
- Total parotidectomy: resection of entire parotid gland (including superficial and deep lobes) usually with preservation of the facial nerve.

BACKGROUND

Intraoperative EMG nerve monitoring can be used as an adjunct to identify and preserve cranial nerves. Facial nerve monitoring has been shown to be cost-effective in middle ear and mastoid surgery; the American Academy of Otolaryngology has approved a position statement regarding its use in otologic surgery.[10,11] In contrast, there has been conflicting data on the effectiveness of facial nerve monitoring during parotid surgery to reduce iatrogenic injury. Because of the paucity of high-level studies with most published data consisting of retrospective reviews, it has not been possible to draw definitive conclusions or develop a formal clinical practice guideline on the indications for facial nerve monitoring during parotidectomy. However, there are current studies that suggest that intraoperative facial nerve monitoring can be helpful in certain situations. The applications, outcomes, and trends with respect to facial nerve monitoring are reviewed in this article.

DISCUSSION
Applications of Facial Nerve Monitoring

Intraoperative EMG nerve monitoring can be used in parotid surgery to identify the facial nerve and follow its course. Although nerve monitoring cannot substitute for anatomic knowledge or skill, it can be helpful in situations where a tumor or previous surgery distort the normal anatomy, precluding the use of standard landmarks. In addition, peripheral nerve branching is variable and unique between patients, and intraoperative monitoring allows for mapping where extensive dissection may be required. There may be unexpected aberrant anatomy of the facial nerve for which EMG can help confirm neural tissue and distinguish from sensory nerves.[12]

Identification of surgical maneuvers that are possibly detrimental to the nerve is another application of intraoperative EMG. Injury to the nerve can occur through multiple mechanisms including stretch, compression, ischemia, thermal injuries, and transection. Triggered responses during manipulation of the tissues can alert the surgeon to the proximity of the nerve to allow for technical adjustments. An absent response may signify disruption of nerve integrity, which would prompt the surgeon to examine the nerve and potentially repair an injury if identified.

Prognostication of facial nerve function is reported as another benefit of intraoperative monitoring. A study by Harig Haring and colleagues[13] demonstrated that the number of intraoperative mechanical events correlated with postoperative facial nerve function. Elevated postdissection thresholds were also found to be associated with immediate temporary facial nerve weakness. This information can aid in patient counseling. However, false-negative signals can occur related to tissue or fascia over the nerve, blood in the field, misplaced electrodes, or incorrect use of the stimulator. False-positive signals can occur if the nerve is stimulated distal to the site of the injury or if an injury occurs after the last testing stimulation.[13]

Consistent use allows the surgeon and staff to become familiar and comfortable with the monitoring device, which increases the ability to troubleshoot, potentially reducing the false-positive and -negative events. With experience, the surgeon can interpret the sounds from the monitor to differentiate artifacts from true events associated with surgical manipulations around the facial nerve. In academic institutions, routine use also helps train medical students and residents in the use of intraoperative nerve monitoring, which is considered a competency of the American Board of Otolaryngology.[14]

Outcomes of Using Facial Nerve Monitoring

The most feared complication during parotid surgery is facial nerve injury. Factors that can affect facial nerve outcomes include size of the lesion, involvement of the deep lobe, malignant cause, extent of parotidectomy, and primary versus revision setting.

Several prospective and retrospective studies have assessed the use of intraoperative facial nerve monitoring in these different scenarios.

Individual studies comparing outcomes between facial nerve monitoring and unmonitored cases for primary parotidectomy have shown conflicting results. Although a retrospective study of 247 patients by Savaas and colleagues demonstrated a significantly reduced incidence in postoperative facial nerve dysfunction with the use of intraoperative monitoring, a prospective 2-center trial of 100 parotidectomies by Grosheva and colleagues found no difference.[15,16] A systematic review published in 2015 by Sood and colleagues analyzed a total of 546 patients across 7 studies, including the article from Grosheva and colleagues, and found that intraoperative facial nerve monitoring significantly decreased the risk of immediate facial nerve weakness compared with the unmonitored group (22.5% vs 34.9%; $P = .001$)[17]; this did not hold true for the incidence of permanent weakness for which there was no significant difference (3.9% vs 7.1%; $P = .18$).[17] A recent systematic review by Witt and colleagues confirming these findings are summarized in **Table 1** (Witt RL, Asarkar A, Sajisevi M, Goodman JF, Coca K, Enepekides D, Mamidala M, Gillespie, B. Facial Nerve Monitoring During Parotidectomy: A systematic review and consensus statement. JAMA Otolaryngology. 2020 (submitted)). When the primary cases are evaluated by extent of parotidectomy, there is significantly less transient facial nerve paralysis in monitored compared with unmonitored patients in superficial parotidectomy. No significant difference was found for partial superficial parotidectomy and total parotidectomy (Witt RL, Asarkar A, Sajisevi M, Goodman JF, Coca K, Enepekides D, Mamidala M, Gillespie, B. Facial Nerve Monitoring During Parotidectomy: A systematic review and consensus statement. JAMA Otolaryngology. 2020 (submitted)).

Multiple studies assessing facial nerve monitoring in revision parotidectomy show shorter recovery time of transient facial nerve paralysis in monitored patients compared with unmonitored patients.[18,19] Furthermore, the severity of facial weakness was found to be decreased in monitored patients.[18,19] However, the data are conflicting regarding the incidence of temporary and permanent weakness with facial nerve monitoring in revision surgery.[18,19] Operative times were significantly shorter in revision parotidectomy with facial nerve monitoring.[18] These

Table 1
Summary of findings from systematic review and consensus statement by Witt and colleagues evaluating outcomes of facial nerve monitoring during parotidectomy

	Primary Parotidectomy	Revision Parotidectomy
Transient facial nerve paresis	Significantly less transient facial nerve paralysis with monitoring	No significant difference with monitoring
Permanent facial nerve paralysis	No significant difference with monitoring	Data suggest less permanent paralysis with monitoring (not statistically significant)
Severity of facial weakness and facial nerve recovery time	Inconclusive	Significantly shorter recovery time and less severity of weakness in monitored patients
Operative times	No difference with monitoring for partial superficial, superficial, or total parotidectomy	Significantly shorter operative times in monitored patients

findings in revision parotid surgery were corroborated by Witt and colleagues as summarized in **Table 1** (Witt RL, Asarkar A, Sajisevi M, Goodman JF, Coca K, Enepekides D, Mamidala M, Gillespie, B. Facial Nerve Monitoring During Parotidectomy: A systematic review and consensus statement. JAMA Otolaryngology. 2020 (submitted)).

Trends in Facial Nerve Monitoring

Practice variations exist with respect to use of intraoperative facial nerve monitoring during parotid surgery. A published survey of practicing otolaryngologists in 2005 demonstrated that 60% of respondents (869/1445) used facial nerve monitoring some or all of the time.[20] Use of facial nerve monitoring correlated with use during training. The use of facial nerve monitoring also correlated positively with the higher volume surgeons, with 79% more likely to use it if they performed more than 10 parotidectomies per year. There was no statistically significant association between the use of monitoring and a history of inadvertent permanent facial nerve injury. However, surgeons who used monitoring in their practice were 20.8% less likely to have a history of a parotid surgery-associated lawsuit. The most common reasons cited for use of monitoring were to help identify the nerve (20%) and medicolegal reasons (14%). Top reasons against use of intraoperative nerve monitoring included that it was not needed (26%) and reliance on anatomy (19%).

A more recent survey of American Head & Neck Society members in 2020 found an increased proportion of respondents routinely use intraoperative nerve monitoring (Witt RL, Asarkar A, Sajisevi M, Goodman JF, Coca K, Enepekides D, Mamidala M, Gillespie, B. Facial Nerve Monitoring During Parotidectomy: A systematic review and consensus statement. JAMA Otolaryngology. 2020 (submitted)). Out of 271 respondents, 77% report routine use in primary parotidectomy for benign lesions, 80% for malignant tumors, 80% for deep lobe/total parotidectomy, and 96% for revision surgery. Most of the respondents thought there was no overall impact on incidence or severity of transient facial weakness or operative time. There was an almost even split in regard to whether respondents thought facial nerve monitoring reduced permanent weakness, slightly favoring "no" (51% vs 49%). The most common reason cited by the survey for using monitoring was medical-legal concerns (63%) followed by for teaching trainees (55%). A minority of respondents (13%) do not use monitoring. The most common reason cited for not using was that there is no substitute for knowledge of anatomy (20%) followed by unproven benefit (13%).

SUMMARY

Facial nerve injury is the most feared complication during parotid surgery owing to the consequent morbidity. Intraoperative EMG nerve monitoring can be used in parotid surgery to identify the facial nerve, map its course, identify surgical maneuvers that are possibly detrimental to the nerve, and provide prognostic information. Data regarding outcomes with facial nerve monitoring are heterogeneous; however, multiple studies corroborate lower incidence of transient weakness in primary parotidectomy. In contrast, the incidence of permanent weakness has not been shown to be significantly affected by use of nerve monitoring. For revision surgery, monitored patients had weaknesses that were less severe with quicker recoveries and shorter operative times compared with unmonitored patients. There seems to be an increasing proportion of surveyed otolaryngologists who routinely use intraoperative nerve monitoring for parotidectomy.

CLINICS CARE POINTS

- Intraoperative electromyographic nerve monitoring does not substitute for knowledge of anatomy and skill but can be used as an adjunct in parotid surgery to identify the facial nerve and map its course.

- Incidence of temporary weakness is significantly reduced with intraoperative nerve monitoring compared with unmonitored patients in primary parotidectomy.

- Permanent facial nerve paralysis has not been shown to be significantly affected by use of nerve monitoring.

DISCLOSURE

The author has nothing to disclose.

REFERENCES

1. Pinkston JA, Cole P. Incidence rates of salivary gland tumors: results from a population-based study. Otolaryngol Head Neck Surg 1999;120(6):834–40.
2. Laccourreye H, Laccourreye O, Cauchois R. Total conservative parotidectomy for primary benign pleomorphic adenoma of the parotid gland: a 25-year experience with 229 patients. Laryngoscope 1994;104:1487–94.
3. Dell' Aversana Orabona G, Bonavolonta' P, Iaconetta G, et al. Surgical management of benign tumors of the parotid gland: extracapsular dissection versus superficial parotidectomy—our experience in 232 cases. J Oral Maxillofac Surg 2013;71:410–3.
4. Kartush J, Lee A. Intraoperative cranial nerve monitoring. In: Babu, editor. Practical neurotology and skull base surgery. San Diego (CA): Plural publishing Inc; 2013. Chapter 11.
5. Eisner Neuromonitoring in central skull base surgery S. Eisner T Fiegele Cavernous Sinus pp89-104.
6. Delgado TE, Bucheit WA, Rosenholtz HR, et al. Intraoperative monitoring of facial muscle evoked responses obtained by intracranial stimulation of the facial nerve: a more accurate technique for facial nerve dissection. Neurosurgery 1979;4: 418–21.
7. Kartush J, Benscoter B. Intraoperative facial nerve monitoring. In: Guntinas-Lichius, Schaitkin, editors. Facial nerve disorders and diseases: diagnosis and management. Stuttgart (NY): Theime Verlagsgruppe; 2016. p. 200–12.
8. Larian B. Parotidectomy for benign parotid tumors. Otolaryngol Clin North Am 2016;49:395–413.
9. Yu G, Peng X. Conservative and functional surgery in the treatment of salivary gland tumours. Int J Oral Sci 2019;11:22.
10. Wilson L, Lin E, Lalwani A. Cost-effectiveness of intraoperative facial nerve monitoring in middle ear or mastoid surgery. Laryngoscope 2003;113(10):1736–45.
11. Position Statement: Intraoperative Nerve Monitoring in Otologic Surgery. 2017. Available at: https://www.entnet.org/intraoperative-nerve-monitoring. Accessed September 27, 2020.
12. Lee DH, Yoon TM, Lee JK, et al. Facial nerve anomaly in a patient with a parotid tumor. Medicine 2016;95(18):e3601.
13. Harig Haring CT, Ellsperman SE, Edwards BM, et al. Assessment of intraoperative nerve monitoring parameters associated with facial nerve outcome in

parotidectomy for benign disease. JAMA Otolaryngol Head Neck Surg 2019; 145(12):1137–43.

14. American Board of Otolaryngology. 2007. Available at: https://www.aboto.org/pub/Core%20Curriculum.pdf. Accessed September 27, 2020.

15. Savvas E, Hillmann S, Weiss D, et al. Association between facial nerve monitoring with postoperative facial paralysis in parotidectomy. JAMA Otolaryngol Head Neck Surg 2016;142(9):828–33.

16. Grosheva M, Klussmann JP, Grimminger C, et al. Electromyographic facial nerve monitoring during parotidectomy for benign lesions does not improve the outcome of postoperative facial nerve function: a prospective two-center trial. Laryngoscope 2009;119(12):2299–305.

17. Sood AJ, Houlton JJ, Nguyen SA, et al. Facial nerve monitoring during parotidectomy: a systematic review and meta-analysis. Otolaryngol Head Neck Surg 2015; 152(4):631–7.

18. Makeieff M, et al. Continuous facial nerve monitoring during parotid adenoma recurrence surgery. Laryngoscope 2005;115:1310–4.

19. Liu H, Wen W, Huang H, et al. Recurrent pleomorphic adenoma of the parotid gland: intraoperative facial nerve monitoring during parotidectomy. Otolaryngol Head Neck Surg 2014;151(1):87–91.

20. Lowry TR, Gal TJ, Brennan JA. Patterns of use of facial nerve monitoring during parotid gland surgery. Otolaryngol Head Neck Surg 2005;133:313–8.

IgG4-Related Disease and the Salivary Glands

A Review of Pathophysiology, Diagnosis, and Management

S. Andrew Skillington, MD, MSCI, M. Allison Ogden, MD*

KEYWORDS

- IgG4-related disease • Sialadenitis • Salivary glands • Mikulicz • Küttner

KEY POINTS

- IgG4-related disease is a systemic disease with head and neck manifestations, most commonly in the salivary glands.
- Mikulicz's disease and Kuttner's tumor are recognized to be part of the IgG4-related diseases.
- The diagnostic criteria for IgG4-related disease are emerging and require clinical, pathologic, radiologic, and serologic correlations.
- Medical management is the standard treatment for IgG4-related disease, typically with glucocorticoids.
- The role for surgical intervention, such as sialendoscopy, is not well-understood for patients with IgG4-related disease, although there is rationale for benefit in this cohort.

INTRODUCTION

Immunoglobulin G4-related disease (IgG4-RD) is an immune-mediated, systemic disease characterized by elevated serum IgG4 levels, tissue infiltration with lymphocytes, fibrosis, and resultant organ dysfunction.[1,2] IgG4-RD was first described as a disease entity in 2003, when several conditions that were previously thought to be unrelated were shown to occur simultaneously in a proportion of patients.[3] These conditions are now recognized to be part of IgG4-RD and are listed in **Box 1**.[1,2,4] In the years since it was first described, IgG4-RD has been shown to affect virtually any organ in the body, with the salivary glands being among the most frequently involved. In a

The authors do not have any relevant conflicts of interest to disclose.
Department of Otolaryngology–Head and Neck Surgery, Washington University School of Medicine in St. Louis, 660 South Euclid Avenue, PO Box 8115, St Louis, MO 63110, USA
* Corresponding author.
E-mail address: ogdenm@wustl.edu

Box 1
Diseases now recognized to fall within the spectrum of IgG4-related disease

Type I autoimmune pancreatitis (lymphoplasmacytic sclerosing pancreatitis)

Sclerosing cholangitis

Retroperitoneal fibrosis (Ormond's disease)

Hypertrophic pachymeningitis

Mikulicz's disease

Riedel's thyroiditis

Küttner's tumor

Eosinophilic angiocentric fibrosis

Multifocal fibrosclerosis

Inflammatory pseudotumor

Mediastinal fibrosis

Inflammatory aortic aneurysm

Periaortitis and periarteritis

Idiopathic hypocomplementemic tubulointerstitial nephritis with extensive tubulointerstitial deposits

Sclerosing mesenteritis

---

cohort of 493 patients with IgG4-RD, 38% had salivary gland involvement.[5] Therefore, it is important that providers who treat salivary gland diseases have a thorough understanding of the pathophysiology, diagnosis, and management of IgG4-RD. Although the awareness of IgG4-RD has increased, this condition continues to be frequently misdiagnosed as neoplastic, infectious, or other inflammatory diseases.[6,7] This review summarizes the most current knowledge of the pathophysiology, diagnosis, and management of IgG4-RD as it relates to the salivary glands.

PATHOPHYSIOLOGY

Although IgG4-RD can affect any organ, it has predilection for certain organ systems. The major salivary glands, the orbits, the lacrimal glands, the pancreas and biliary tree, the lungs, the kidneys, the aorta and retroperitoneum, the meninges, and the thyroid are most affected.[8] The disease typically follows a biphasic course that is characterized by an initial inflammatory phase followed by a fibrosing outcome.[9]

In the inflammatory phase, polyclonal B and T cell subpopulations infiltrate affected tissues and undergo mutual activating, antigen-mediated interactions leading to the secretion of profibrotic cytokines such as IL-1β, IL-6, interferon-γ, transforming growth factor-β, and platelet-derived growth factor B.[10] Several lymphocyte subpopulations have been implicated including plasmablasts/plasma cells, cytotoxic T lymphocytes, and CD4$^+$ T follicular helper cells.[11,12] Although cytotoxic T lymphocytes have not been shown to induce tissue fibrosis directly, plasmablasts from patients with IgG4-RD have been shown to activate fibroblasts and collagen production in vitro.[13,14] T follicular helper cells play an important role in the inflammatory phase by driving IgG4 class switching, promoting IgG4-committed B-cell clonal expansion, and enhancing the maturation of naïve B cells into mature plasma cells, leading to the production and secretion of IgG4.[15] Currently, the contribution of IgG4 antibodies to the pathogenesis of IgG4-RD is poorly understood, but it has been proposed is that IgG4 antibodies and cytotoxic T lymphocytes act synergistically to induce tissue inflammation.[16]

In the second, fibrosing phase of the disease, innate immune cells, such as M2 macrophages, infiltrate IgG4-RD lesions and secrete profibrotic cytokines including IL-10, IL-13, and IL-33.[17] Activated fibroblasts begin to deposit extracellular matrix, resulting in a dense stromal reaction that distorts the tissue, architecture leading to organ dysfunction and possibly organ failure.[9]

EPIDEMIOLOGY

Because IgG4-RD is a newly recognized entity, its incidence and prevalence are not established. The majority of IgG4-RD epidemiologic studies have been conducted in Japan focusing on type I autoimmune pancreatitis. The prevalence of type I autoimmune pancreatitis in Japan is estimated at 2.2 cases per 100,000.[18] However, because the pancreas is only one of many possible organs that can be involved, this would be an underestimation of the prevalence of IgG4-RD. Men are disproportionately affected, which contrasts starkly from many other autoimmune diseases.[1,2] The ratio of men to women is about 2:1 and most patients present in their 50s or 60s.[5] How the prevalence of IgG4-RD varies across ethnicities and race has not been investigated thoroughly, but Asians and Caucasians seem to be affected disproportionately.[5] Currently, there are no environmental or genetic risk factors clearly associated with IgG4-RD.[4]

CLINICAL PRESENTATION

Because IgG4-RD can affect a wide range of organ systems, the clinical presentation is diverse. Patients present with symptoms related to the affected organ systems. In general, the onset of IgG4-RD is subacute; thus, patients are not constitutionally ill.[2] About 75% of patients have multiorgan involvement; however, because the affected organs may have subclinical involvement, multiorgan disease can evolve over time.[2,5] IgG4-RD is often associated with allergic disease. Patients may present with elevated IgE levels and peripheral eosinophilia.[19] About 40% to 44% of patients with IgG4-RD have a history of allergic disease including allergic rhinitis, asthma, urticaria, eczema, and hypersensitivity pneumonitis.[19,20]

In patients with salivary gland involvement, isolated, bilateral submandibular gland enlargement is the most common presentation; however, the parotid glands and sublingual glands are also frequently enlarged with associated tenderness.[1,2] Minor salivary glands can be affected, even if macroscopically normal in appearance.[1,2] Xerostomia is frequently present but not as severe as seen in Sjögren's syndrome.[1] Sialolithiasis, salivary stasis, and mucous plugs are possible and are secondary to sialadonitis.[21]

Although IgG4-RD has only recently been recognized as a disease entity, 2 previously described salivary gland diseases—namely, Mikulicz's disease and Küttner's tumor—are now known to fall under the spectrum of IgG4-RD.[1,2] In 1888, Johann von Mikulicz-Radecki first reported a case of a farmer who presented with bilateral submandibular, parotid, and lacrimal gland swelling.[22] Mikulicz described tumor like growths of all glands with benign lymphoid tumors on histology.[22] This constellation of findings became known as Mikulicz's disease, later being called benign lymphoepithelial lesion.[23] In 1896, Hermann Küttner first described a condition characterized by firm, nodular swelling isolated to 1 or both submandibular glands.[24] This disease became known as Küttner's tumor or chronic sclerosing sialadenitis.[25] Mikulicz's disease and Küttner's tumor are both included in IgG4-RD, yet the 2 entities have different clinical presentations. These differences are highlighted in **Table 1**.[21,26]

CLINICAL PHENOTYPES

In 2019, Wallace and colleagues[5] identified 4 distinct clinical phenotypes of IgG4-RD using a latent class analysis of 493 patients with IgG4-RD disease. This study was the first to group patients with IgG4-RD with an otherwise diverse clinical presentation into mutually exclusive, homogeneous groups based on organ involvement. The characteristics of the 4 phenotypes are presented in **Table 2**. The first group is typified by pancreatohepatobiliary involvement. The second group is typified by aortic and retroperitoneal involvement. The third group is limited to head and neck disease in a pattern of incomplete Mikulicz. The fourth group is characterized by head and neck disease in a pattern more consistent with Mikulicz's disease, along with widespread systemic involvement. Of note, the third group is significantly more likely to be younger, female, and Asian when compared with the other 3 groups. The fourth group has significantly higher serum IgG4 levels. The second group has significantly lower serum IgG4 levels. Although each IgG4-RD phenotype has a unique distribution of organ involvement, it is important to note that the salivary glands can be affected in any phenotype.[5] The clinical and treatment implications of the phenotype designations are yet to be fully determined.

DIAGNOSIS

IgG4-RD mimics many neoplastic, infectious, and inflammatory diseases; thus, the diagnosis can be challenging. Establishing the appropriate diagnosis requires the correlation of clinical, radiologic, serologic, and pathologic data. When considering a diagnosis of IgG4-related sialadenitis, other important diagnostic considerations include Sjögren's syndrome, sarcoidosis, lymphoma, and sialodocholithiasis.[1,2]

Pathology

In 2011, at the First International Symposium on IgG4-RD, a consensus statement based on expert opinion was released that aimed to provide pathologists with diagnostic guidelines.[27] This consensus statement on the pathology of IgG4-RD identified 5 histopathologic hallmarks of IgG4-RD: dense lymphoplasmacytic infiltrate, tissue fibrosis with a "storiform" pattern, obliterative phlebitis, infiltrating IgG4+ plasma cells, and an IgG4+ to IgG+ plasma cell ratio exceeding 40% on immunohistochemistry

Table 1
Variability in clinical presentation between Mikulicz's disease and Küttner's tumor

	Mikulicz's Disease	Küttner's Tumor
Organ involvement	Lacrimal, submandibular, and parotid glands	Submandibular glands only
Laterality and symmetry	Bilaterally symmetric	Unilateral or bilaterally asymmetric
Gland appearance	Diffuse, smooth swelling	Nodular, firm swelling
Sialoliths, salivary stasis, or mucous plugs	Not observed	Frequently present

Table 2
Clinical phenotypes of IgG4-related disease

	Group I, Pancreatohepatobiliary	Group II, Retroperitoneum/Aorta	Group III, Head and Neck Limited	Group IV, Mikulicz/Systemic
Predominant organ involvement	Pancreas, liver, biliary tree	Retroperitoneum, aorta	Orbit, lacrimal glands, salivary glands, sinuses	Lacrimal glands, salivary glands, sinuses, pancreas, biliary tree, kidneys, lungs, lymph nodes, prostate
Age	Older	Older	Younger	Older
Gender	Male	Male	Female	Male
Race	White	White	Asian	Equivocal
Serum IgG4	Elevated	Normal to mildly elevated	Elevated	Profoundly elevated

(**Fig. 1**). The first 3 histopathologic features are essential to establish a diagnosis of IgG4-RD. Although the presence of IgG4+ plasma cells and a high IgG4+ to IgG+ plasma cell ratio both support the diagnosis of IgG4-RD, these findings are nonspecific because they are found in many inflammatory and neoplastic conditions. Additionally, the extent of IgG4+ plasma cell tissue infiltrate in IgG4-RD varies depending on the affected organ. Fine needle aspiration biopsies may not be sufficient to identify the morphologic features of IgG4-RD; a core, incisional, or excisional biopsy should be considered if further evaluation is indicated. Pathologic features such as tissue necrosis, granulomas, leukocytoclastic vasculitis, or neutrophils are not characteristic of IgG4-RD, thereby indicating an alternative diagnosis.[27]

Within the salivary glands, histopathologic features of IgG4-RD include preserved lobular architecture and large lymphoid follicles with hypercellular germinal centers occupying the gland parenchyma.[28–30] In contrast with Sjögren's syndrome, the salivary ducts remain largely spared without lymphocytic infiltration and only mild acinar destruction.[28,29] Two of the histopathologic hallmarks of IgG4-RD—namely, storiform fibrosis and obliterative phlebitis—are inconsistently observed in the salivary glands, being more common in retroperitoneal, pancreatic, and biliary lesions.[29,30] Therefore, the diagnosis of IgG4-related sialadenitis based on histopathologic criteria is not always straightforward; clinical, radiographic, and serologic correlation is required.

Serology

Elevated serum IgG4 is a characteristic finding of IgG4-RD, yet this marker is neither sensitive nor specific for IgG4-RD. It is elevated in about 50% to 90% of patients. The degree of serum IgG4 elevation correlates with the severity of disease and the number of organs involved.[31,32] In a meta-analysis of 9 case control studies that included 1235 patients with IgG4-RD and 5696 controls, the serum IgG4 upper limit of normal ranged from 135 to 144 mg/dL. Using this upper limit of normal as a cutoff, an elevated serum IgG4 provided a sensitivity of 87% and specificity of 83% for the diagnosis of IgG4-

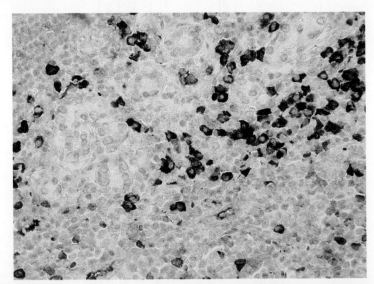

Fig. 1. Submandibular gland histology demonstrating IgG4+ plasma cell infiltration [100x, IgG4 Immunostain]. (*Courtesy of* M. Boyd Gillespie, MD, Memphis, TN.)

RD.[33] Using a cutoff of twice the upper limit of normal (270–280 mg/dL) provided increased specificity (95%) at the cost of decreased sensitivity (63%).[33] Thus, the serum IgG4 level is informative, but it is not accurate as a stand-alone diagnostic test. Serum IgG1, IgG2, IgG3, and total IgG are also often elevated in IgG4-RD but not to the extent of IgG4.[32,34,35] The ratio of serum IgG4 to serum total IgG has been proposed as a diagnostic marker; however, this metric has shown poorer diagnostic accuracy than serum IgG4 alone.[36]

Coinciding with the frequently observed elevated serum IgG4 levels, mild hyperproteinemia may be present about one-half of the time in IgG4-RD.[35] Additionally, polyclonal hypergammaglobulinemia on serum protein electrophoresis has been reported in 37% to 80% of cases.[34,35] Complement consumption with low serum C3 and C4 concentrations has been reported in 14% to 56% of patients with active IgG4-RD.[32,34,35] In these patients, it is important to check a urinalysis, because complement consumption is associated with subclinical or overt renal involvement.[32] Antinuclear antibodies are sometimes present in low titers, but disease-specific autoantibodies such as antineutrophil cytoplasmic antibody, anti-Ro/SS-A, anti-La/SS-B, and anti-dsDNA are not found in IgG4-RD.[34,35]

Serologic markers of inflammation such as the erythrocyte sedimentation rate and C-reactive protein may be elevated in IgG4-RD, but are nonspecific markers. About one-half of patients have a moderately elevated erythrocyte sedimentation rate.[32,34] CRP is also elevated in about one-half of patients but is particularly associated with IgG4-RD with aortic/periaortic involvement.[32,34,37] Atopy is associated with IgG4-RD in about 30% to 44% cases.[19,20,34,38] Accordingly, elevated concentrations of serum IgE is present in 35% to 67% of cases. Eosinophilia is identified in about one-third of cases.[19,32,34,35,38]

Radiology

Radiologic studies alone generally cannot establish a diagnosis of IgG4-RD, but can provide useful ancillary data.[1,2] IgG4-related autoimmune pancreatitis is the exception. Computed tomography (CT) scans and MRI classically show a diffusely enlarged pancreas with a capsule-like rim, no ductal dilatation, and without a low-density mass.[39] These findings can be diagnostic of IgG4-related autoimmune pancreatitis in the appropriate clinical setting.[39] In contrast, imaging findings in IgG4-related sialadenitis are nonspecific. CT scans and MRI show diffusely enlarged major salivary glands without other significant findings.[30,40] In some cases, superficial enhancement of the parotid glands may be present.[40] This finding is in contrast to Sjögren's syndrome, which characteristically shows a "salt-and-pepper" appearance on CT scans and MRI.[40] Doppler ultrasound examination is the imaging modality of choice in IgG4-related sialadenitis in showing highly vascular nodal and reticular patterns specific to IgG4-RD in comparison with Sjögren's syndrome.[40] A PET scan with fludeoxyglucose/CT scan typically shows abnormal FDG uptake in salivary glands affected by IgG4-RD; however, this modality has poor specificity.[40] A PET scan with fludeoxyglucose/CT scan is most useful for IgG4-RD in staging and evaluating treatment response.[41]

Diagnostic Guidelines

Multiple consensus statements and guidelines have been published to assist clinicians in accurately diagnosing IgG4-RD. The current diagnostic criteria were established in 2011 at the First International Symposium on IgG4-RD.[42] These criteria classify IgG4-RD as definitive, probable, or possible based on clinical, serologic, and pathologic data. When pathologic confirmation is not available, a possible diagnosis of IgG4-RD can be provided.[42]

More recently, a system for classifying IgG4-RD was proposed by the American College of Rheumatology and European League Against Rheumatism.[43] In 2019, an international, multidisciplinary group of 86 physicians developed and validated a classification criteria for IgG4-RD based on more than 1000 cases of IgG4-RD and nearly 800 cases of mimicker diseases. These classification criteria consist of a 3-step process. First, there must be characteristic involvement either clinically, radiologically, or pathologically of at least 1 of 10 typical organs. Second, numerous clinical, serologic, radiologic, and pathologic exclusion criteria must be absent. Finally, additional weighted inclusion criteria are scored and summed. If the cumulative score is 20 or higher, then the patient meets the classification criteria. The aim of this classification system was to identify homogeneous groups of patients with IgG4-RD for research purposes. Indeed, this algorithm has shown a very high specificity for IgG4-RD (98%) with an acceptable sensitivity (82%).[43] Although not developed as a diagnostic tool, this system has shown usefulness as a diagnostic framework promising to become widely adopted.[4]

MANAGEMENT

Treatment for IgG4-RD depends on the severity of disease, affected organ systems, and individual patient factors. IgG4-RD is generally much more responsive to treatment during the early inflammatory phase than the later fibrotic phase when irreversible organ damage has occurred.[44] IgG4-RD often follows a relapsing–remitting course.[45] Therefore, it is important to consider both the initial treatment regimen as well as long-term maintenance therapy.

Glucocorticoids

Glucocorticoids are the first-line treatment in all patients with active IgG4-RD.[45] Generally, patients respond rapidly to medium or high-dose steroids within days to weeks.[45] If patients show no response to steroids, the diagnosis of IgG4-RD should be questioned because IgG4-RD is characteristically steroid responsive.[45] The duration of treatment is highly variable, but current guidelines suggest continuing the initial steroid dose for 2 to 4 weeks before tapering over the course of 3 to 6 months.[45] Faster tapering or early discontinuation is associated with a higher rate of relapse.[46]

Immunosuppressants

Numerous traditional immunosuppressants have been used to treat IgG4-RD, yet there is a paucity of evidence to support their use. Methotrexate, azathioprine, mycophenolate mofetil, leflunomide, tacrolimus, cyclosporin A, cyclophosphamide, and iguratimod have all been used in combination with corticosteroids to induce remission.[45,47] These immunosuppressants are administered in conjunction with corticosteroids as a part of the initial treatment regimen when there are concerning disease features such as multiorgan involvement or high serum IgG4 levels.[45] A meta-analysis of 15 observational studies showed that dual immunosuppressant and steroid therapy was superior in achieving remission when compared with steroids or immunosuppressants alone.[47] Additionally, there may be a role for traditional immunosuppressants among patients with contraindications to corticosteroids. However, this approach has not been investigated thoroughly.

Biologic Agents

Rituximab was the first and remains the most widely used biologic agent for IgG4-RD.[48] Rituximab can be used in combination with corticosteroids to induce disease remission and allow early corticosteroid tapering.[48] Perhaps the most important role of rituximab in IgG4-RD is in maintenance therapy. Rituximab is more effective at preventing relapses than other traditional immunosuppressants; however, its dosing and administration protocols are not clearly established in this setting.[47] Multiple other biologic agents have been used in isolated, refractory cases of IgG4-RD, such as abatacept, infliximab, and dupilumab, but their role in treating IgG4-RD is not well-defined.[4]

Surgical Intervention

Because IgG4-RD is a systemic disease characteristically highly responsive to medical management, surgical intervention is not a standard treatment protocol.[45] Excisional or incisional biopsy can be used for diagnostic purposes. Further roles of surgery have not been fully investigated for IgG4-RD sialadenitis. To our knowledge, there are no reported case series of patients with IgG4-RD treated with sialendoscopy or salivary endoscopy. Sialendoscopy has the potential to treat IgG4-related sialadenitis by removing sialoliths and debris, dilating stenotic ducts, and infiltrating corticosteroid medications, as has been shown to have usefulness in management of other autoimmune diseases.[26]

SUMMARY

IgG4-RD is a relatively recently defined systemic disease, often affecting salivary glands. Patient presentation, evaluation, and treatment typically occurs across disciplines, thus requiring recognition and understanding in various surgical and medical fields to adequately diagnose and manage affected patients. Further study is needed to determine how medical management of IgG4-RD can be augmented by surgical techniques, such as sialendoscopy, to maximize patient outcomes.

CLINICS CARE POINTS

- The diagnosis of Immunoglobulin G4 – Related Disease (IgG4-RD) affecting the salivary glands requires clinical correlation; radiographic, serologic and pathologic analyses; and a high-index of suspicion.
- Salivary IgG4-RD manifests as gland swelling or enlargement, with possible associated pain and/or dry mouth.
- The strict diagnostic criteria for IgG4-RD are emerging and used most readily for research purposes.
- IgG4-RD is treated with systemic glucocorticoids, with or without other immunosuppressants.
- Surgery is typically reserved for diagnosis, excisional or incisional biopsy.
- Sialendoscopy can be considered for symptoms or signs of sialadenitis in the setting of IgG4-RD.

REFERENCES

1. Kamisawa T, Zen Y, Pillai S, et al. IgG4-related disease. Lancet 2015;385(9976): 1460–71.
2. Stone JH, Zen Y, Deshpande V. IgG4-related disease. N Engl J Med 2012;366(6): 539–51.

3. Kamisawa T, Funata N, Hayashi Y, et al. A new clinicopathological entity of IgG4-related autoimmune disease. J Gastroenterol 2003;38(10):982–4.

4. Lanzillotta M, Mancuso G, Della-Torre E. Advances in the diagnosis and management of IgG4 related disease. BMJ 2020;369:m1067.

5. Wallace ZS, Zhang Y, Perugino CA, et al. Clinical phenotypes of IgG4-related disease: an analysis of two international cross-sectional cohorts. Ann Rheum Dis 2019;78(3):406–12.

6. Lanzillotta M, Campochiaro C, Trimarchi M, et al. Deconstructing IgG4-related disease involvement of midline structures: comparison to common mimickers. Mod Rheumatol 2017;27:638–45.

7. Carruthers R, Carruthers M, Della-Torre E. IgG4-related disease and other causes of inflammatory meningeal disease. Semin Neurol 2014;34:395–404.

8. Stone JH, Khosroshahi A, Deshpande V, et al. Recommendations for the nomenclature of IgG4-related disease and its individual organ system manifestations. Arthritis Rheum 2012;64:3062–7.

9. Pillai S, Perugino C, Kaneko N. Immune mechanisms of fibrosis and inflammation in IgG4-related disease. Curr Opin Rheumatol 2020;32:146–51.

10. Della-Torre E, Feeney E, Deshpande V, et al. B-cell depletion attenuates serological biomarkers of fibrosis and myofibroblast activation in IgG4-related disease. Ann Rheum Dis 2015;74:2236–43.

11. Della-Torre E, Bozzalla-Cassione E, Sciorati C, et al. A CD8α subset of CD4+SLAMF7+ cytotoxic T cells is expanded in patients with IgG4-related disease and decreases following glucocorticoid treatment. Arthritis Rheumatol 2018; 70:1133–43.

12. Mattoo H, Mahajan VS, Della-Torre E, et al. De novo oligoclonal expansions of circulating plasmablasts in active and relapsing IgG4-related disease. J Allergy Clin Immunol 2014;134:679–87.

13. Della-Torre E, Rigamonti E, Perugino C, et al. B lymphocytes directly contribute to tissue fibrosis in patients with IgG4-related disease. J Allergy Clin Immunol 2020; 145:968–81.

14. Mattoo H, Mahajan VS, Maehara T, et al. Clonal expansion of CD4(+) cytotoxic T lymphocytes in patients with IgG4-related disease. J Allergy Clin Immunol 2016; 138:825–38.

15. Chen Y, Lin W, Yang H, et al. Aberrant expansion and function of follicular helper T cell subsets in IgG4-related disease. Arthritis Rheumatol 2018;70:1853–65.

16. Sasaki T, Yajima T, Shimaoka T, et al. Synergistic effect of IgG4 antibody and CTLs causes tissue inflammation in IgG4-related disease. Int Immunol 2020;32: 163–74.

17. Furukawa S, Moriyama M, Tanaka A, et al. Preferential M2 macrophages contribute to fibrosis in IgG4-related dacryoadenitis and sialoadenitis, so-called Mikulicz's disease. Clin Immunol 2015;156:9–18.

18. Kanno A, Nishimori I, Masamune A, et al. Nationwide epidemiological survey of autoimmune pancreatitis in Japan. Pancreas 2012;41(6):835–9.

19. Kamisawa T, Anjiki H, Egawa N, et al. Allergic manifestations in autoimmune pancreatitis. Eur J Gastroenterol Hepatol 2009;21(10):1136–9.

20. Liu Y, Xue M, Wang Z, et al. Salivary gland involvement disparities in clinical characteristics of IgG4-related disease: a retrospective study of 428 patients. Rheumatology (Oxford) 2020;59(3):634–40.

21. Kamiński B, Błochowiak K. Mikulicz's disease and Küttner's tumor as manifestations of IgG4-related diseases: a review of the literature. Reumatologia 2020; 58(4):243–50.

22. Mikulicz J. In: Billroth T, editor. Über eine eigenartige symmetrische erkränkung der thränen—und mundspeicheldrüsen. Stuttgart (Germany): Beiträge zur Chir Festschrift Gewidmet Stuttgart Ger Ferdinand Enke; 1892. p. 610–30.
23. Penfold CN. Mikulicz syndrome. J Oral Maxillofac Surg 1985;43(11):900–5.
24. Küttner H. Über entzündliche tumoren der submaxillar-speicheldrüse. Beitr Klin Chir 1896;15:815–34.
25. Uhliarova B, Svec M. Küttner tumor. Bratisl Lek Listy 2013;114(1):36–8.
26. Gallo A, Martellucci S, Fusconi M, et al. Sialendoscopic management of autoimmune sialadenitis: a review of the literature. Acta Otorhinolaryngol Ital 2017;37(2): 148–54.
27. Deshpande V, Zen Y, Chan JK, et al. Consensus statement on the pathology of IgG4-related disease. Mod Pathol 2012;25:1181–92.
28. Moriyama M, Furukawa S, Kawano S, et al. The diagnostic utility of biopsies from the submandibular and labial salivary glands in IgG4-related dacryoadenitis and sialoadenitis, so-called Mikulicz's disease. Int J Oral Maxillofac Surg 2014;43: 1276–81.
29. Umehara H, Okazaki K, Masaki Y, et al. A novel clinical entity, IgG4-related disease (IgG4RD): general concept and details. Mod Rheumatol 2012;22:1–14.
30. Li W, Chen Y, Sun ZP, et al. Clinicopathological characteristics of immunoglobulin G4-related sialadenitis. Arthritis Res Ther 2015;17(1):186.
31. Carruthers MN, Khosroshahi A, Augustin T, et al. The diagnostic utility of serum IgG4 concentrations in IgG4-related disease. Ann Rheum Dis 2015;74(1):14–8.
32. Wallace ZS, Deshpande V, Mattoo H, et al. IgG4-related disease: clinical and laboratory features in one hundred twenty-five patients. Arthritis Rheumatol 2015; 67(9):2466–75.
33. Hao M, Liu M, Fan G, et al. Diagnostic value of serum IgG4 for IgG4-related disease: a PRISMA-compliant systematic review and meta-analysis. Medicine (Baltimore) 2016;95(21):e3785.
34. Campochiaro C, Ramirez GA, Bozzolo EP, et al. IgG4-related disease in Italy: clinical features and outcomes of a large cohort of patients. Scand J Rheumatol 2016;45:135–45.
35. Ebbo M, Daniel L, Pavic M, et al. IgG4-related systemic disease: features and treatment response in a French cohort: results of a multicenter registry. Medicine (Baltimore) 2012;91(1):49–56.
36. Yang H, Li J, Wang Y, et al. Distribution characteristics of elevated serum immunoglobulin G4 (IgG4) and its relationship with IgG4-related disease. Scand J Rheumatol 2019;48(6):497–504.
37. Akiyama M, Kaneko Y, Takeuchi T. Characteristics and prognosis of IgG4-related periaortitis/periarteritis: a systematic literature review. Autoimmun Rev 2019; 18(9):102354.
38. Della Torre E, Mattoo H, Mahajan VS, et al. Prevalence of atopy, eosinophilia, and IgE elevation in IgG4-related disease. Allergy 2014;69(2):269–72.
39. Shimosegawa T, Chari ST, Frulloni L, et al. International consensus diagnostic criteria for autoimmune pancreatitis: guidelines of the International Association of Pancreatology. Pancreas 2011;40(3):352–8.
40. Shimizu M, Okamura K, Kise Y, et al. Effectiveness of imaging modalities for screening of IgG4-related dacryoadenitis and sialadenitis (Mikulicz's disease) and for differentiating it from Sjögren's syndrome (SS), with an emphasis on sonography. Arthritis Res Ther 2015;17:223.
41. Ebbo M, Grados A, Guedi, et al. Usefulness of 2-[18F]-fluoro-2-deoxy-D-glucose-positron emission tomography/computed tomography for staging and evaluation

of treatment response in IgG4-related disease: a retrospective multicenter study. Arthritis Care Res 2014;66:86–96.

42. Umehara H, Okazaki K, Masaki Y, et al. Comprehensive diagnostic criteria for IgG4-related disease (IgG4-RD), 2011. Mod Rheumatol 2012;22(1):21–30.

43. Wallace ZS, Naden RP, Chari S, et al. The 2019 American College of Rheumatology/European League Against Rheumatism classification criteria for IgG4-related disease. Ann Rheum Dis 2020;79(1):77–87.

44. Zhang WSJ, Stone JH. Management of IgG4-related disease. Lancet Rheumatol 2019;1:e55.

45. Khosroshahi A, Wallace ZS, Crowe JL, et al. Second International Symposium on IgG4-Related Disease. International consensus guidance statement on the management and treatment of IgG4-related disease. Arthritis Rheumatol 2015;67: 1688–99.

46. Kubota K, Kamisawa T, Okazaki K, et al. Low-dose maintenance steroid treatment could reduce the relapse rate in patients with type I autoimmune pancreatitis: a long-term Japanese multicenter analysis of 510 patients. J Gastroenterol 2017; 52:955–64.

47. Omar D, Chen Y, Cong Y, et al. Glucocorticoids and steroid sparing medications monotherapies or in combination for IgG4-RD: a systematic review and network meta-analysis. Rheumatology (Oxford) 2020;59(4):718–26.

48. Khosroshahi A, Carruthers MN, Deshpande V, et al. Rituximab for the treatment of IgG4-related disease. Medicine (Baltimore) 2012;91:57–66.

SURGICAL TECHNIQUES

Incorporating Sialendoscopy into the Otolaryngology Clinic

Christopher D. Badger, MD, MBA*, Daniel A. Benito, MD,
Arjun S. Joshi, MD

KEYWORDS

• Sialendoscopy • Sialolithiasis • Sialadenitis • Salivary glands • In-office

KEY POINTS

- Sialendoscopy may be successfully performed in the outpatient clinic with careful patient selection.
- This practice decrease the financial burden, time, and anesthesia required for treatment without an increase in complications.
- Those wishing to incorporate sialendoscopy into their outpatient clinic should first become comfortable with sialendoscopy in the operating room.
- An outpatient sialendoscopy practice may be built gradually by beginning with the simplest diagnostic cases and gradually adding interventional cases with experience.
- Diagnostic endoscopy, dilation of stenosis, and endoscopic sialolithotomies of small, mobile stones are techniques well-suited for in-office sialendoscopy.

BACKGROUND

Advances in technology and equipment have led to an increasing number of salivary procedures being performed in the clinic under local anesthesia in lieu of in the operating room. When these procedures are selected carefully, they offer patients efficient and convenient treatment of salivary disorders without the added burden and potential risks associated with general anesthesia in the operating room. Sialendoscopy, both as a diagnostic and therapeutic intervention, is well-suited to the otolaryngologist's clinic. With experience, preparation, and proper equipment, sialendoscopy may be performed safely in the clinic with few complications. In-office sialendoscopy procedures are associated with a decreased procedure time and financial burden when compared with procedures performed in the operating room.[1]

Since sialendoscopy was first described by Katz in 1991 for the use of salivary gland exploration and stone extraction using miniaturized basket catheters, it has been used

Division of Otolaryngology–Head & Neck Surgery, George Washington University School of Medicine & Health Sciences, 2300 M. Street, 4th Floor, Washington, DC 20037, USA
* Corresponding author.
E-mail address: cbadger@mfa.gwu.edu

Otolaryngol Clin N Am 54 (2021) 509–520
https://doi.org/10.1016/j.otc.2021.02.003
oto.theclinics.com

to evaluate the ductal system for the identification of obstructions and stricture of the duct through direct visualization.[2] Francis Marchal and his colleagues[3,4] significantly advanced the field with their development of the instruments and techniques that are commonly used today. In particular, the development of the semirigid endoscope with a working channel has allowed sialendoscopy to flourish. Despite being described by Marchal and colleagues as a procedure that can be performed under local anesthesia in the office, many otolaryngologists in North America continue to perform sialendoscopy in the operating room. Although it is reasonable to perform complicated cases that may require conversion to a more extensive surgical approach in the operating room, many pathologies are accessible and treatable via an endoscopic or transoral approach under local anesthesia in the otolaryngology clinic. Over the last 10 years, the senior author has performed nearly 1000 sialendoscopy procedures in the clinic with relatively few major or minor complications (data to be published). The procedure is generally well-tolerated by patients who are grateful for being spared the financial burden, time cost, and risks of general anesthesia.

Despite these benefits, successfully incorporating sialendoscopy into the clinic requires judgment and experience in selecting cases best suited to the clinic or the operating room. It is our recommendation that the otolaryngologist wishing to incorporate sialendoscopy into the outpatient clinic first gain experience with the procedure in the operating room before introducing it to the outpatient clinic. This process allows the otolaryngologist to gain experience with the technique and identify cases appropriate for in-office sialendoscopy.

EVALUATION

Although the value of sialendoscopy for the evaluation of ductal pathologies cannot be overstated, the authors begin the evaluation of salivary gland swelling with the history, physical examination, and ultrasound examination at the initial visit. The use of surgeon-performed ultrasound examinations is helpful in identifying the extent of the pathology, and frequently offers a clear diagnosis at the initial visit, negating the need for further diagnostic imaging in the radiology department.[5,6] Salivary ultrasound serves as an extension of the physical examination in the hands of an experienced head and neck surgeon. It is sensitive and specific (96.6% and 90.0%, respectively) for the detection of salivary stones when combined with sonopalpation by an experienced otolaryngologist.[7] Furthermore, ultrasound examination may be used to assess the size of sialoliths accurately and determine their orientation in the duct.[8] The widely cited algorithm proposed by Marchal and Dulguerov[9] proposes that stones less than 4 mm for the submandibular gland, or less than 3 mm for the parotid gland, are amenable to extraction through sialendoscopy via a wire basket without the need for lithotripsy. However, the work by Walvekar and colleagues[10] has demonstrated that stones larger than the cutoffs established by Marchal and colleagues may be amenable to endoscopic extraction if oriented favorably with their largest dimension in the length of the duct. Nevertheless, ultrasound examination provides a quick, noninvasive assessment that may be useful when deciding if sialendoscopy is appropriate or clinically useful. Furthermore, the information gained from an ultrasound examination can aid the surgeon when selecting the setting for sialendoscopy.

CONTRAINDICATIONS

The only relative contraindication to sialendoscopy is acute sialadenitis. Not only is sialendoscopy more difficult during acute infection, but instrumentation to the inflamed duct may increase the risk of ductal trauma or perforation. Furthermore, mucopurulent saliva may hamper visualization on endoscopy.

INDICATIONS

Given the dual roles of sialendoscopy as a diagnostic and therapeutic modality, it is indicated for the treatment and evaluation of a number of salivary pathologies. The main use of sialendoscopy is for the evaluation of ductal pathologies. The primary indications for sialendoscopy are to evaluate obstructive sialolithiasis, ductal stricture, salivary swelling of unclear origin, and intraductal masses.

Salivary Gland Swelling of Unclear Origin

Given the semi-invasive nature of sialendoscopy, the author prefers to reserve diagnostic sialendoscopy for the evaluation of salivary gland swelling of unclear origin after an initial evaluation with salivary ultrasound, preferably performed by an experienced head and neck surgeon. Despite the accuracy of an ultrasound examination, up to 5% of cases remain unclear after an ultrasound examination, as well as a computed tomography scan or MRI.[11] These cases usually show indirect signs of obstruction, such as intraglandular dilation, main ductal dilation, and sialectasis without a definite stone, stenosis, or other obstruction. In a retrospective study by Koch and colleagues,[11] 103 patients with chronic swelling of the major glands of unclear origin underwent sialendoscopy. Stenosis or obstruction by fibrotic plugs was the most common abnormality (56.6%), followed by sialolithiasis (20.3%), dochitis (10.7%), and anatomic malformation (3.9%). Only 10.7% of these patients demonstrated normal findings.[11]

Obstructive Sialadenitis

Sialolithiasis remains the most common cause of obstructive sialadenitis.[4,12,13] In-office sialendoscopy is well-suited for the extraction of small, mobile sialoliths using a wire basket. Lithotripsy may be used to remove larger or impacted concretions; however, the authors recommend the use of a nonendoscopic open approach for extraction or reserving cases requiring lithotripsy for the operating room. This caution is due to the increase in time, equipment, and patient discomfort associated with these larger stones. Extracorporeal shockwave lithotripsy, intracorporeal laser fragmentation lithotripsy, and pneumatic lithotripsy are options for the endoscopic removal of larger sialoliths; however, the lack of regulatory approval in parts of the world, including North America, has limited its widespread use.

Ductal stenosis or stricture is the second most common cause of benign salivary gland obstruction.[14–18] Sialendoscopy is an ideal method for the diagnosis of ductal stenoses. It allows for the direct visualization of stenoses to assess the location, severity, length, and number of stenoses.[19] Additionally, sialendoscopy with ductal dilation is the preferred treatment method for stenosis. Various techniques may be used for stenosis, including mechanical methods such as balloon, bougie, or sialendoscope, and transoral sialodochoplasty ductal marsupialization, as well as hydrostatic techniques such as the instillation of saline or steroids. These techniques to treat stenosis may all be performed in the clinic with practice.

Mucous plugging is a common cause of obstructing sialadenitis. It is often seen in cases of sialolithiasis, Sjogren's syndrome, juvenile recurrent parotitis, and radioiodine-induced sialadenitis. These plugs may serve as a nidus for eventual stone formation.[20,21] Mucous plugging can be washing out the obstruction with saline irrigation.

Obstructive sialadenitis owing to a foreign body is an infrequent but established cause of sialopathy. Human hair, wood, feathers, pen caps, pencil lead, metal staples, fish bones, and glass have been documented in the literature.[22,23]

PATIENT COUNSELING

Patients should be counseled to expect some mild discomfort and swelling of the gland as the anesthetic and saline irrigation are injected into the ductal tree. In-office sialendoscopy is generally well-tolerated by patients. However, it is helpful to ask about the patient's tolerance of dental procedures to gauge their level of comfort with a transoral procedure. If dental procedures were poorly tolerated, consideration should be given to performing sialendoscopy under general anesthesia. A small dose of oral alprazolam may be given as an anxiolytic before the procedure. Additionally, an oral pain medication such as an opiate may be administered. Patients should be counseled regarding aggravation of temporomandibular joint disorders; however, having the patient awake may mitigate excessive oral opening by maintaining muscular tone and allowing for awake patient feedback. Patients should also be counseled regarding the risk of iatrogenic obstructions owing to scarring and stenosis associated with instrumentation. This complication is generally prevented by careful technique with close interval follow-up after the initial procedure.

TECHNIQUE
Preparation

A mayo stand is prepared with the listed equipment (**Box 1**, **Fig. 1**). The sialendoscope is connected to light source, camera, and 0.9% NaCl IV bag outfitted with tubing, a syringe, and a stopcock or 3-way valve (**Fig. 2**). The patient is comfortably seated upright in the examination chair.

Cannulation

In-office sialendoscopy begins by injecting the mucosa surrounding the affected papilla with 1% lidocaine with 1:100,000 epinephrine (**Fig. 3**). The papilla is then identified and confirmed by passing a 0.015-inch diameter by 50-cm long fixed core titanium guide wire into the papilla (**Fig. 4**). Gentle massage on the affected gland can aid in the identification of the papilla as saliva is milked from the gland (**Fig. 5**).[24] A sialagogue, such as a citric acid powder, may be applied to stimulate salivation and further aid in the identification of the papilla. A Seldinger technique is used to dilate the papilla by passing a flexible salivary access dilator over the wire (**Fig. 6**).[25] The senior author generally begins with the 5F salivary access dilator, because the conical tip allows for atraumatic dilation of the duct, and the outer diameter (1.7 mm) allows for sufficient dilation for passage of the sialendoscope while minimizing the need for subsequent serial dilation. Gentle irrigation with a few milliliters of the chosen anesthetic is then performed through the dilator, not through the sialendoscope side port. A 2% viscous lidocaine may be used in place of traditional lidocaine with epinephrine (**Fig. 7**). This agent helps to stent open the duct during sialendoscopy and requires less irrigation during the diagnostic portion of sialendoscopy. If mucous plugging is suspected, the senior author prefers traditional lidocaine instillation because this substance allows for better irrigation of mucinous collections. Anesthesia of the ductal tree develops over several minutes after ductal infusion. The dilator may remain in the affected papilla during this time to aid in subsequent papilla identification.

Immediately before cannulation with the sialendoscope (**Fig. 8**), the dilator is removed for sialendoscope insertion. Sialendoscope insertion may also be performed

Box 1
In-office sialendoscopy basic equipment

Telescope
- 1.1 or 1.3 mm all-in-one sialendoscope
  - Light source
  - Camera

Irrigation
- IV pole with 250 mL 0.9% NaCl saline and tubing with stopcock or 3-way valve
- 10-mL syringe

Anesthetic
- 1% Lidocaine with 1:100,000 epinephrine
- Optional: Viscous lidocaine oral topical solution 2%

Surgical instruments
- Cheek retractor
- Conical dilator
- Lacrimal probes
- Toothed forceps
- Hemostat
- Scissors

Disposables
- 50-cm Fixed core wire guide (straight)
- Salivary access dilator set (4F, 5F, 6F, and7F)

Optional
- Wire basket

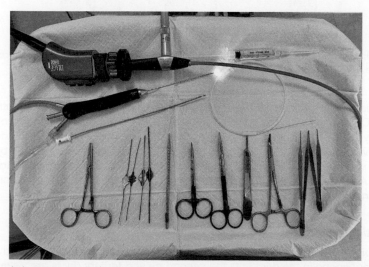

Fig. 1. Basic instruments and equipment. A mayo tray is set up with a 1.1 mm "all-in-one" sialendoscope attached to a camera, light source, and saline irrigation. The tray contains a hypodermic syringe with local anesthetic (1% lidocaine with 1:100,000 epinephrine), various hemostats, a needle driver, scissors, lacrimal probes, conical dilator, guide wire, and salivary access dilator.

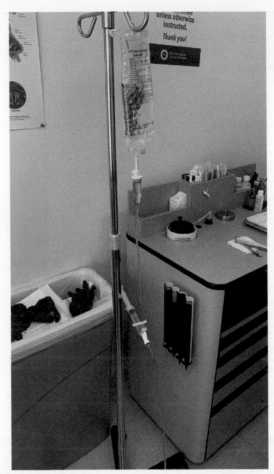

Fig. 2. Saline irrigation. IV pole with 250 mL 0.9% NaCl saline and tubing with stopcock or 3-way valve.

via a Seldinger technique, but is often unnecessary once the papilla is sufficiently dilated. Once the ductal lumen is visualized via the introduced sialendoscope, the duct may be gently explored. The sialendoscope may be atraumatically advanced as small volumes of saline irrigation are injected by an assistant. Care should be taken to avoid overirrigating the duct. Increased hydrostatic pressure may lead to ductal rupture. A sufficient volume should be used to allow facilitate ductal opening and advancement of the sialendoscope proximally.

Diagnostic Sialendoscopy

At this point, the diagnostic portion of sialendoscopy is performed by gently advancing the sialendoscope in the duct until the secondary and tertiary ducts are visualized or the offending obstruction is identified. Diagnostic sialendoscopy is ideal for diagnosing ductal pathologies including stenosis, dilatation, and sialolithiasis. It is particularly useful when direct signs of sialolithiasis, such as hyperechoic lines or acoustic shadowing, are absent on ultrasound examination, but indirect signs of obstruction

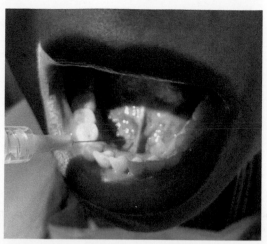

Fig. 3. Submucosal injection of local anesthetic: 1% lidocaine with 1:100,000 epinephrine is injected submucosally in the area surrounding the affected papilla.

are present, such as intraglandular dilation, main ductal dilation, and sialectasis.[7] In such cases, the sialendoscope may clarify the clinical picture by identifying sialoliths too small to be seen on ultrasound examination or a computed tomography scan. Additionally, the sialendoscope may be used to identify and characterize stenotic patterns within the salivary duct. The most common classification system used is Marchal's LSD classification system.[26,27] The 3 components of this classification system, lithiasis (L), stenosis (S), and dilation (D), characterize the ductal pattern of salivary disease. The presence or absence of stones should be identified. If present, the stone should be identified as either free floating or fixed. An estimate of its size should be made. The location of the stone and whether the stone is palpable with a gloved finger should also be noted. This procedure will help the practitioner to decide between endoscopic sialolithotomy, transoral sialolithotomy, or a hybrid approach. Likewise, the nature of any identified stenosis may be characterized by intraductal diaphragmatic stenosis (S1), an isolated main ductal stenosis (S2), multiple or diffuse main

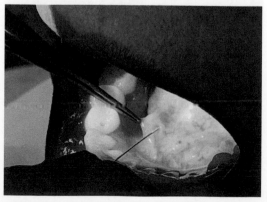

Fig. 4. Cannulation of the duct. A 50-cm fixed core titanium guide wire is passed into the papilla to canulate the duct.

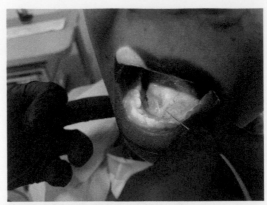

Fig. 5. Identification of the papilla. Gentle massage of the affected gland may help to identify the papilla as saliva is milked through the duct.

ductal stenosis (S3), or generalized stenosis involving the main and intraglandular ducts (S4). Dilation is similarly classified as involving a single isolated dilated segment (D1), multiple dilated segments (D2), or generalized with involvement of the entire ductal tree (D3).[27] These observations will aid the practitioner when planning future interventions.

Ductal Dilation

Ductal dilation may be offered to patients with evidence of symptomatic ductal obstruction caused by ductal stenosis after ruling out sialolithiasis. This procedure should be performed after the stenotic segment is visualized on endoscopy. This procedure may be performed using a balloon, bougie, rigid dilator, saline hydrodilation, or the endoscope itself. The simplest of these techniques is saline hydrodilation. In many cases, hydrodilation may allow for sufficient dilation of a stenotic segment without the need and the risks associated with more aggressive instrumentation. As always, the authors recommend accounting for the patient's comfort level, procedure length, and degree of instrumentation when selecting cases for the clinic. Hydrodilation may be safely performed in most in-office sialendoscopies with a relatively low risk.

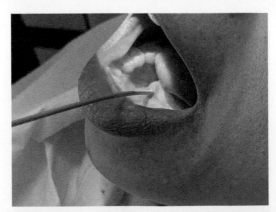

Fig. 6. Dilation. A flexible salivary access dilator is passed over the guide wire into the duct to dilate the papilla. The guide wire is then removed in preparation for instilling local anesthetic into the ductal tree.

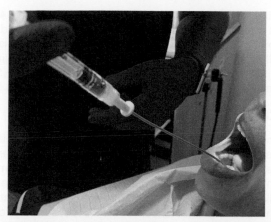

Fig. 7. Instillation of anesthetic into the ductal system. Anesthetic is instilled into the ductal system through the access dilator using 1% lidocaine with 1:100,000 epinephrine or viscous lidocaine. The dilator may remain in the affected papilla until the sialendoscope is passed into the duct.

Endoscopic Sialolithotomy

Endoscopic sialolithotomy may be performed in the clinic; however, the authors reserve this technique for small free-floating stones without distal stenoses. A wire basket is used to retrieve the stones; however, the practitioner should be prepared in the event the stone and basket become impacted at the papilla as the stone is withdrawn. This situation may be addressed with a distal dochotomy at the papilla to facilitate stone extraction. However, it is better to prevent impaction of the stone and wire basket by carefully assessing the diameter of the ductal lumen and papilla distal to the stone. If the distal duct or papilla is stenotic, this may be the root cause preventing spontaneous passage of the sialolith. In these cases, the patient is better served by a procedure that alleviates the distal narrowing such as transoral sialolithotomy and sialodochoplasty to extract the stone and prevent future impaction. Transoral surgical sialolithotomy performed in the office may be offered as a viable alternative to

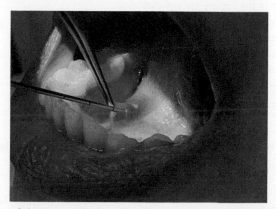

Fig. 8. Cannulation of the duct with the sialendoscope. The sialendoscope is passed through the dilated papilla and the ductal lumen is visualized.

endoscopic sialolithotomy for submandibular stones larger than 4 mm or parotid stones larger than 3 mm[9] to minimize the risk of distal impaction during extraction. If the patient is comfortable with an oral procedure and the stone is easily palpated in the floor of mouth, consideration should be given to transoral sialolithotomy and sialodochoplasty. This procedure addresses directly the obstructing stone and widens the distal duct to allow for spontaneous passage of sialoliths in the future.

POSTOPERATIVE CARE

After sialendoscopy, the patient should be counseled to continue with copious hydration, sialagogue use, and milking of the salivary gland. In cases where a sialodochotomy was performed, the patient should return 1 week later to confirm ductal patency. A lacrimal probe may be passed through the sialodochoplasty to confirm patency and provide gentle dilation. It is the senior author's experience that this procedure adequately prevents scarring and stenosis of the duct secondary to instrumentation and papillotomy. Restenosis and obstruction of the duct are rare in those seen 1 week later with patency confirmed by lacrimal probe. In some cases, patients who underwent sialodochotomy and experience symptom recurrence over the 7 days after their procedure have been spared a repeat sialodochotomy by performing a gentle dilation with lacrimal probe at this follow-up visit.

SUMMARY

Diagnostic sialendoscopy and simple interventional sialendoscopy techniques may be performed in the otolaryngology clinic with few complications. This procedure is generally well-tolerated by patients and decreases the time, financial burden, and anesthesia required for sialendoscopy. Incorporating sialendoscopy into the otolaryngology clinic should begin after sialendoscopy experience is gained in the operating room. Simple techniques such as diagnostic sialendoscopy, endoscopic sialolithotomy of small mobile stones, and hydrodilation of stenotic segments are generally appropriate for the otolaryngology clinic. Patient anxiety and comfort should be considered when identifying cases appropriate for the otolaryngology clinic.

CLINICS CARE POINTS

- Diagnostic sialendoscopy, simple dilations, and sialolithotomy of small mobile stones may be safely performed in the otolaryngology clinic.
- The selection of cases for in-office sialendoscopy should depend on patient comfort, anatomy, and type of salivary pathology.
- Sialendoscopy performed in the otolaryngology clinic is safe, convenient, and cost-effective with thoughtful patient selection

DISCLOSURE

The authors have no relevant financial relationships or conflicts of interest to disclose.

REFERENCES

1. Coniglio AJ, Deal AM, Bhate O, et al. In-office versus operating room sialendoscopy: comparison of outcomes, patient time burden, and charge analysis. Otolaryngol Head Neck Surg 2019;160(2):255–60.

2. Katz P. Endoscopy of the salivary glands. Ann Radiol 1991;34:110–3. Available at: https://pubmed.ncbi.nlm.nih.gov/1897843/. Accessed August 24, 2020.
3. Marchal F, Becker M, Dulguerov P, et al. Interventional sialendoscopy. Laryngoscope 2000;111(1):2427–9.
4. Marchal F, Dulguero P, Lehmann W, et al. Submandibular diagnostic and interventional sialendoscopy: new procedure for ductal disorders. Ann Otol Rhinol Laryngol 2002;111(1):27–35.
5. Goncalves M, Mantsopoulos K, Schapher M, et al. Ultrasound supplemented by sialendoscopy: diagnostic value in sialolithiasis. Otolaryngol Head Neck Surg 2018. https://doi.org/10.1177/0194599818775946.
6. Benito DA, Badger C, Hoffman HT, et al. Recommended imaging for salivary gland disorders. Curr Otorhinolaryngol Rep 2020. https://doi.org/10.1007/s40136-020-00299-2.
7. Patel NJ, Hashemi S, Joshi AS. Sonopalpation: a novel application of ultrasound for detection of submandibular calculi. Otolaryngol Head Neck Surg (United States 2014;151(5):770–5.
8. Badger CD, Patel S, Romero NJ, et al. In vivo accuracy of ultrasound for sizing salivary ductal calculi. Otolaryngol Neck Surg 2020. https://doi.org/10.1177/0194599820937676. 019459982093767.
9. Marchal F, Dulguerov P. Sialolithiasis management: the state of the art. Arch Otolaryngol Head Neck Surg 2003;129(9):951–6.
10. Walvekar RR, Carrau RL, Schaitkin B. Endoscopic sialolith removal: orientation and shape as predictors of success. Am J Otolaryngol Head Neck Med Surg 2009;30(3):153–6.
11. Koch M, Zenk J, Bozzato A, et al. Sialoscopy in cases of unclear swelling of the major salivary glands. Otolaryngol Head Neck Surg 2005;133(6):863–8.
12. Marchal F, Dulguerov P, Becker M, et al. Specificity of parotid sialendoscopy. Laryngoscope 2001;111(2):264–71.
13. Rice DH. Noninflammatory, non-neoplastic disorders of the salivary glands. Otolaryngol Clin North Am 1999;32(5):835–42.
14. Ngu RK, Brown JE, Whaites EJ, et al. Salivary duct strictures: nature and incidence in benign salivary obstruction. Dentomaxillofac Radiol 2007;36(2):63–7.
15. Koch M, Zenk J, Iro H. Diagnostic and interventional sialoscopy in obstructive diseases of the salivary glands. HNO 2008;56(2):139–44.
16. Yu C, Yang C, Zheng L, et al. Endoscopic observation and strategic management of obstructive submandibular sialadenitis. J Oral Maxillofac Surg 2010;68(8): 1770–5.
17. Chuangqi Y, Chi Y, Lingyan Z. Sialendoscopic findings in patients with obstructive sialadenitis: long-term experience. Br J Oral Maxillofac Surg 2013;51(4): 337–41.
18. Lee LIT, Pawar RR, Whitley S, et al. Incidence of different causes of benign obstruction of the salivary glands: retrospective analysis of 403 cases using fluoroscopy and digital subtraction sialography. Br J Oral Maxillofac Surg 2015; 53(1):54–7.
19. Koch M, Zenk J, Iro H. Stenosis and stenosis-like lesions in the submandibular duct: detailed clinical and sialendoscopy-based analysis and proposal for a classification. Oral Surg Oral Med Oral Pathol Oral Radiol 2020. https://doi.org/10.1016/j.oooo.2020.05.015.
20. Marchal F, Kurt AM, Dulguerov P, et al. Retrograde theory in sialolithiasis formation. Arch Otolaryngol Head Neck Surg 2001;127(1):66–8.

21. Harrison JD. Causes, Natural History, and Incidence of Salivary Stones and Obstructions. Otolaryngol Clin North Am 2009;42(6):927–47.
22. Gill AS, Kieliszak CR, Joshi AS. Sialendoscopy as a management tool in patients with foreign body impaction of the salivary gland. Am J Otolaryngol Head Neck Med Surg 2016;37(4):369–71.
23. Sreetharan SS, Philip R. Unusual foreign body of parotid gland presenting as sialolithiasis: case report and literature review. Case Rep Otolaryngol 2012; 2012:1–3.
24. Kent DT, Walvekar RR, Schaitkin BM. Sialendoscopy: getting started, how long does it take? Laryngoscope 2016;126(5):1083–5.
25. Chossegros C, Guyot L, Richard O, et al. A technical improvement in sialendoscopy to enter the salivary ducts. Laryngoscope 2006;116(5):842–4.
26. Myers EN, Ferris RL. Salivary Gland Disorders. 2007. https://doi.org/10.1007/978-3-540-47072-4.
27. Marchal F, Chossegros C, Faure F, et al. Salivary stones and stenosis. A comprehensive classification. Rev Stomatol Chir Maxillofac 2008;109(4):233–6.

Open Approaches to Stensen Duct Scar

Leighton F. Reed, MD[a], M. Boyd Gillespie, MD, MSc[a], Trevor Hackman, MD[b],*

KEYWORDS

- Stensen duct • Salivary duct • Salivary duct scar • Salivary duct stricture
- Salivary duct stenosis • Salivary duct repair • Chronic sialadenitis

KEY POINTS

- Salivary duct scar (Stenosis [circumferentially narrowed duct]; Sticture [scar blockage of lumen]) is the second most common cause of obstructive sialadenitis after stone.
- Stensen duct is the duct most prone to scar formation.
- First-line gland-preserving treatment includes dilation using endoscopic techniques.
- Open duct repair using end-to-end anastomosis or vein interposition grafting is an option for patients who fail endoscopic intervention or who have severe or complex stenoses.

BACKGROUND

Salivary duct scarring typically originates in the setting of general glandular inflammation. It may have multiple etiologies, including stone, trauma, autoimmune disease, and chronic infection. An estimated 50% of cases of obstructive sialadenitis are due to ductal scarring, with the remaining 50% caused by stones. A typical patient presents with glandular swelling and pain during meals or gland stimulation with failure to visualize a stone on follow-up imaging. Performing ultrasonography after sialogogue stimulation often reveals glandular congestion and a dilated visible duct that can be traced distally to a site of obstruction. Salivary duct scar typically consists of either a ductal stenosis or a ductal stricture. Salivary duct stenoses are circumferential, segmental narrowings with a duct diameter less than 1.5 mm that maintain at least partial lumen patency throughout the area of scarring. Ductal stricture is a complete scar blockage extending across the ductal lumen.

DIAGNOSIS

The original method used to diagnosis salivary duct scar was sialography, which had several limitations, including patient discomfort, potential contrast dye allergy, and

[a] Department of Otolaryngology-Head and Neck Surgery, University of Tennessee Health Science Center, 910 Madison Avenue, Suite 408, Memphis, TN 38163, USA; [b] Department of Otolaryngology-Head and Neck Surgery, UNC Hospitals, 170 Manning Drive, Chapel Hill, NC 27599-7070, USA
* Corresponding author.
E-mail address: trevor_hackman@med.unc.edu

Otolaryngol Clin N Am 54 (2021) 521–530
https://doi.org/10.1016/j.otc.2021.01.005
0030-6665/21/© 2021 Elsevier Inc. All rights reserved.

lack of ability to provide real-time therapeutic intervention. Although still useful as a means of creating a 2-dimensional picture of the ductal anatomy, due to the scarcity of providers skilled in sialography and the growing number of skilled sialoendoscopists, sialography largely has been surpassed by sialendoscopy as a diagnostic modality. Sialendoscopy provides intraluminal visualization and characterization of ductal scar while allowing potential therapeutic intervention. The grading system for characterizing duct stenosis proposed by Koch and colleagues[1] achieved via diagnostic sialendoscopy includes a description of the location, length, and grade of the stenosis. The location should be described with reference to the distance from the ostium as well as the anatomic segment (ostium, distal main duct, proximal main duct, hilum, or intraglandular duct). The length of the stenoses should be described as short (<1 cm), intermediate (1–3 cm), or diffuse stenosis (>3 cm or multiple segments).[1] Lastly, the grade is determined by the degree of lumen patency. Tracheal stenosis grading is a convenient rule of thumb familiar to otolaryngologists useful in describing the grade of salivary duct stenosis (grade I = 0–50% stenosis; grade II = 50%–70% stenosis; grade III = 70%–99% stenosis; and grade IV = 100% stenosis). An estimate of lumen patency can be achieved quickly and easily by comparing scope diameter to intraluminal diameter. The Erlangen Salivary Scope System (Storz; Tuttlingen, Germany) has scope diameters of 0.8 mm, 1.1 mm, and 1.6 mm. If comparing to a normal duct lumen of 2.0 mm to 2.5 mm, inability to pass the 0.8-mm scope means a stenosis of greater than 66%, the 1.1-mm scope means greater than 50% stenosis, and the 1.6-mm scope means greater than 33% stenosis. Although there are multiple scope systems, familiarity with the sizes of the system used by a surgeon's institution can provide quick and easy grading estimates.

MANAGEMENT OPTIONS

The parotid duct is responsible for 75% of all salivary duct stenosis.[2] Most of these cases are amenable to minimally invasive gland-preserving therapy with sialendoscopy via a purely endoscopic retrograde approach. Recurrent or higher-grade stenosis involving longer segments of the duct, however, may require more invasive intervention. For more complex cases, a combined approach employing retrograde endoscopic evaluation with ultrasound-guided interventions, such as guided balloon dilations or guided percutaneous transfacial access to allow for anterograde endoscopy or treatment of the stenotic area, also may be successful. The high-grade strictures associated with complete duct obstruction require more invasive open approaches for segmental resection of the involved area, akin to the surgical algorithm escalation for management of tracheal stenoses.[3] High-grade stenoses typically occur secondary to previous surgical procedures of the parotid duct or surrounding tissues or are secondary to local abscess formation.[3] When an open surgical approach is required, surgical techniques that have been described include duct resection with primary end-to-end anastomosis and microvascular vein graft repair.

Open surgical approaches with primary anastomosis of Stensen duct following traumatic laceration is the most extensively characterized approach described in the literature. Comparison of this literature to open surgical approaches for parotid duct stenosis may prove valuable. In trauma evaluation, the duct is categorized into 3 anatomic segments.[4] Site A refers to injuries proximal to the posterior border of the masseter muscle. Site B refers to the duct as it passes over the masseter, and site C is anterior to the masseter. Site A injuries only require closure of the lacerated parotid capsule because the ducts in this location are small and either scar down or recannulate.[5,6] When site B injuries are identified, primary anastomosis is the treatment of choice when possible. The proximal and distal stumps should be dissected from surrounding tissue in order to reduce the tension on the anastomosis.[6,7] An intraductal catheter may be used to assist in approximation by maintaining the lumen of the duct. It is recommended that the catheter remain in place for 2 weeks to prevent stenosis of the anastomotic site.[6,8] Site C injuries also may undergo primary anastomosis, but this is a more difficult procedure because the duct interdigitates with fibers of the superficial muscular aponeurotic system (SMAS). If not feasible, the alternative is reimplantation of the duct with creation of a neo-ostium more posteriorly in the buccal cavity.[5,6] In this scenario, the neo-ostium often is prone to recurrent stricture, given the circular nature of the incision and the contractile forces pulling the duct into the buccal space. Therefore, these patients require regular follow-up with repeated in-office dilation of the neo-ostium as required to maintain patency. When considering open repair of Stensen duct stenosis, the trauma literature provides general guidelines for stenotic repair. Site B and, to a lesser extent, site C are feasible regions for primary anastomosis due to the larger caliber duct and the improved exposure without encasing glandular tissue. After resection of the stenotic duct, primary anastomosis is a viable option if there is sufficient length on the proximal and distal ductal segments to allow a tension-free anastomosis.

After resection of the stenotic duct, primary anastomosis may not be feasible due to excessive tension or inability to approximate the duct orifices. In these scenarios, autogenous vein grafts are an interposition option. The use of autogenous vein grafts in dogs has been studied with conflicting results.[9,10] Subsequently, Özgenel and Özcan[11] investigated the use of autologous vein grafts taken from the cephalic vein to relocate Stensen duct for the treatment of 4 patients with sialorrhea secondary to cerebral palsy. The subjective results of this study may be invalid because the surgery was in conjunction with submandibular rerouting. There were, however, no postoperative complications and no sign of obstruction or stricture at any follow-up visit. This lack of postoperative obstruction or stricture suggests viability of using interposition autogenous vein grafts as a treatment option. In a case report by Heymans and colleagues,[5] an interposition vein graft taken from the antebrachial vein was used successfully for anastomosis after 2 cm of the parotid duct from site B was missing after a traumatic injury. Six months after reconstruction, sialography demonstrated patency of the reconstructed duct. Each study successfully harvested vein grafts from the forearm, including the cephalic and antebrachial veins. An alternative technique may involve fileting the stenosis and using the vein as a patch to re-establish the lumen. Although vessel choice may be patient-specific, the correct size match between forearm vein and the parotid duct in these studies suggest the forearm as an appropriate initial donor site for autogenous vein grafting. In addition, there are numerous potential veins within the surgical field that may be of the proper size, including the facial, external jugular, and retromandibular veins.

Unfortunately, there is a paucity of literature describing open surgical approaches for the correction of Stensen duct stenosis; studies on duct reconstruction after traumatic injury may correlate well and provide a general set of guidelines for patients requiring invasive intervention. The anatomic location of the stenosis may suggest the viability of a successful open surgical approach with ideal locations being site B lesions and to lesser extent site C lesions. If located in a viable location, the ability to achieve a tension-free reconstruction determines whether the optimal surgical choice is primary anastomosis versus interposition vein grafting.

CASE PRESENTATION

A 67-year-old woman with numerous medical comorbidities, including a history of stage III chronic kidney disease status post–renal transplant, presented to clinic with a 21-year history of chronic recurrent right parotid swelling without infections. Her symptoms began suddenly during lunch one day. She was treated with antibiotics, which resolved the presumed infection. Over the subsequent decades, the patient reported persistent recurrent, noninfectious episodes of right parotid swelling. Within the 5 years prior to the authors' evaluation, the patient reported a gradually enlarging, visible, linear, semicylindrical swelling under the skin of the right cheek. When she performed vigorous massage, she could force a large volume of saliva into the mouth, but over the past year, the gland had become more difficult and painful to decompress. In addition, the volume of saliva buildup required her to decompress her gland 5 to 6 times each meal. On initial examination, she was found to have visible convex deformity of the right cheek skin due to a 4-cm dilated segment of parotid duct, which measured 1 cm in diameter on ultrasound.

Given the presence of saliva flow by patient's history and examination, she initially was treated with in-office endoscopy under local anesthesia. The patient's right Stensen duct was evaluated with the 1.1-mm sialendoscope, and a severe grade III stenosis (>70%) was visualized on endoscopy 2.5 cm from the orifice in site B (**Fig. 1**). Simultaneous ultrasonography confirmed the position of the scope abutting the short grade III stenosis and a markedly dilated proximal duct just beyond the stenosis. After placing a guide wire through the stenosis, a balloon catheter was placed over the guide wire using the Seldinger technique and inflated. The balloon was removed and the repeat endoscopy confirmed successful dilation of the stenosis.

Unfortunately, the patient developed recurrent symptoms 6 months later, requiring repeat sialendoscopy. At the subsequent sialendoscopy, the stenosis had worsened in caliber, pliability, and length (now 1 cm based on ultrasound evaluation of the length from the distal portion of the dilated proximal segment and the position of the lacrimal probe tip in the distal duct). Repeat attempts at dilation did not achieve significant improvement. In addition, the patient was counseled that to achieve symptom resolution, the markedly dilated duct would require volume reduction to prevent the buildup of high viscosity saliva, whose increased resistance to clearance would impair salivary outflow regardless of distal duct patency. The authors, therefore, proposed an open

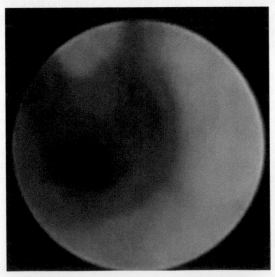

Fig. 1. Endoscopic view of grade III stenosis prior to balloon dilation.

approach to resect a 2.5-cm area of high-grade stenosis and dilated parotid duct in the hopes of restoring the continuity of flow and reduce saliva pooling.

The patient was scheduled for a parotidectomy approach for open treatment of duct stenosis with vein graft repair. A modified Blair incision was designed (**Fig. 2**) and a #0 lacrimal probe was placed into the right Stensen duct orifice and positioned under ultrasound guidance against the stenotic segment. After standard sterile preparation and drape technique, a supra-SMAS flap was elevated anteriorly to the buccal space and the dilated parotid duct and stenotic distal segment in site B (identified by palpation of the lacrimal probe) were isolated (**Fig. 3**). In order to address both the stricture and the ductal dilation, a 2.5-cm segment of duct was resected (**Figs. 4** and **5**). A guide wire was advanced through the distal duct segment from the buccal mucosa orifice into the surgical wound (**Fig. 6**) and serial dilations were performed with Seldinger technique until a 16-gauge angiocathether was advanced successfully through the distal duct over the guide wire into the field (**Fig. 7**). In the neck, a 2.5-cm segment of facial vein, devoid of valves, was isolated and harvested and then brought into the parotid field loaded on a lacrimal probe (**Fig. 8**). Under operative microscope, 8-0 Ethilon suture was used to anastomose the facial vein to the proximal and distal remnant duct segments over the 16-gauge angiocatheter, which then was secured to the buccal mucosa with 4-0 Prolene suture. The parotid incision was closed in standard fashion with deep sutures and tissue sealant. Patient was placed in a jaw bra and sent home with follow-up in 2 weeks.

At the first postoperative appointment, the catheter stent was removed and office sialendoscopy confirmed patency of the vein conduit. Endoscopy revealed patent anastomosis site and expected endothelial shedding and debris in the vein conduit. A second catheter stent was placed and secured to the buccal mucosa with 4-0 Prolene suture for 2 additional weeks. At the subsequent appointment, the stent was removed and the patient was discharged with instructions for hydration and gland massage. At 6 months postprocedure, endoscopy revealed a patent vein conduit (**Fig. 9**). After 18 months of follow-up, she remains free of recurrent obstruction episodes. She still performs twice-daily massage but denies prandial symptoms, swelling, or pain.

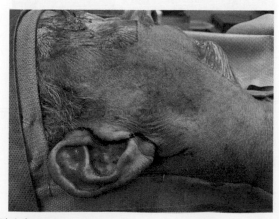

Fig. 2. Modified Blair incision.

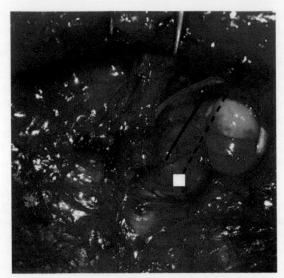

Fig. 3. Parotid duct. The dilated and stenotic segments of duct lay within the solid and dotted black lines.

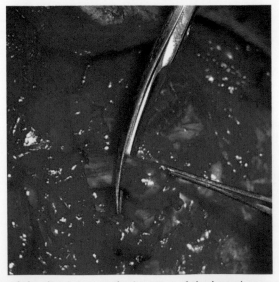

Fig. 4. Transection of the distal duct at the junction of the buccal space.

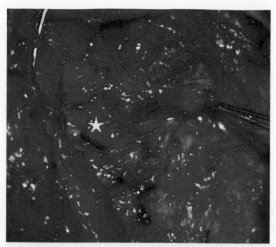

Fig. 5. Transected parotid duct. In this view, the forceps are retracting the distal portion of the proximal duct. On the left of the screen, the lacrimal probe can be seen entering the surgical wound through the remnant distal duct (*star*).

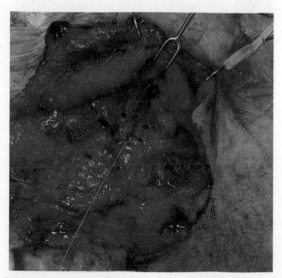

Fig. 6. Transoral placement of the guidewire into the surgical field.

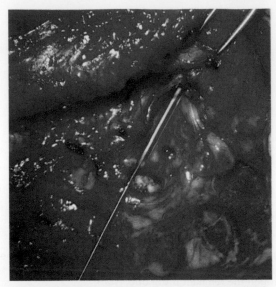

Fig. 7. Seldinger technique for placement of a 16-gauge angiocathether as an indwelling stent entering the surgical field from the oral cavity.

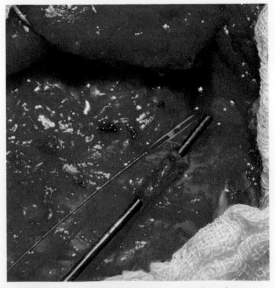

Fig. 8. Vein graft brought into the field over a #0 lacrimal probe.

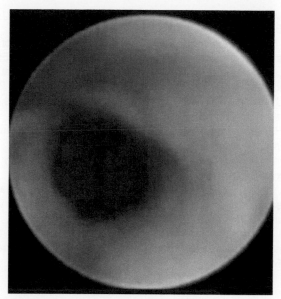

Fig. 9. Appearance of vein conduit 6 months after repair.

CLINICS CARE POINTS

- Tracheal stenosis grading is a useful and familiar scale for grading salivary duct stenosis.
- Minimally invasive gland preserving therapy is first-line treatment, but recurrent or higher-grade stenosis my require more invasive intervention.
- Location of the stenosis determines if an open approach may be considered. Stenoses in site B and select site C cases are amenable to stenosis resection and anastomosis.
- Open approaches for Stenson duct stenosis resection require either primary end-to-end anastomosis or vein interposition grafting with a goal of a tension-free anastomosis.
- Serial in-office endoscopic evaluations and postoperative stenting of the parotid duct for 2 or more weeks after reconstructive surgery are critical for maintaining long-term successful patency of the drainage system.

DISCLOSURE

None.

REFERENCES

1. Koch M, Iro H, Zenk J. Sialendoscopy-based diagnosis and classification of parotid duct stenoses. Laryngoscope 2009;119(9):1696–703.
2. Ngu R, Brown J, Whaites E, et al. Salivary duct strictures: nature and incidence in benign salivary obstruction. Dentomaxillofac Radiol 2007;36(2):63–7.
3. Koch M, Iro H. Parotid gland intraoral/external combined approaches for strictures. In: Wiit RL, editor. Surgery of the salivary gland. Philadelphia: Elsevier Inc; 2021. p. 191–9.

4. Van Sickels JE, Alexander JM. Parotid duct injuries. Oral Surg Oral Med Oral Pathol 1981;52(4):364–7.
5. Heymans O, Nélissen X, Médot M, et al. Microsurgical Repair of Stensen's Duct Using an Interposition Vein Graft. J Reconstr Microsurg 1999;15(02):105–7.
6. Lazaridou M, Iliopoulos C, Antoniades K, et al. Salivary gland trauma: a review of diagnosis and treatment. Craniomaxillofac Trauma Reconstr 2012;5(4):189–95.
7. Steinberg MJ, Herréra AF. Management of parotid duct injuries. Oral Surg Oral Med Oral Pathol Oral Radiol Endodontol 2005;99(2):136–41.
8. Stevenson JH. Parotid duct transection associated with facial trauma: experience with 10 cases. Br J Plast Surg 1983;36(1):81–2.
9. Dumpis J, Feldmane L. Experimental microsurgery of salivary ducts in dogs. J Cranio Maxillofac Surg 2001;29(1):56–62.
10. Özgenel GY, Özcan M, Kahveci Z. An experimental study of bilateral repositioning of the Stensen's duct orifices with autologous vein and artery grafts in dogs. Br J Plast Surg 2000;53(2):106–8.
11. Özgenel GY, Özcan M. Bilateral parotid-duct diversion using autologous vein grafts for the management of chronic drooling in cerebral palsy. Br J Plast Surg 2002;55(6):490–3.

Transoral Excision of Parapharyngeal Space Tumors

Andrew R. Larson, MD[a],*, William R. Ryan, MD[b]

KEYWORDS

- Parapharyngeal space tumors • Salivary neoplasm • Salivary tumors
- Transoral surgery • Transoral robotic surgery • TORS • Endoscope-assisted surgery
- Minimally invasive

KEY POINTS

- Transoral robotic surgery and endoscope-assisted transoral surgery are helpful adjuncts that can enhance exposure and delivery of parapharyngeal space (PPS) masses approached transorally.
- With the advent of these technological advancements, indications for transoral removal of PPS masses have expanded to include larger tumors and those with lateral or poststyloid extension or location.
- When considering a transoral approach to removing a PPS mass preoperatively, a surgeon should consider multiple patient and tumor factors, including, but not limited to, cytopathology, lateral and superior extent of tumor, tumor relationship to the carotid artery, and any patient trismus or limitation in neck flexion/extension.
- For a large or lateral-extending PPS tumor, transcervical assistance through a 2.5- to 4-cm neck incision may be used to facilitate tumor mobilization and transoral tumor delivery.
- Transoral PPS tumor excisions can eliminate the risk of first bite syndrome and a neck incisional scar.

INTRODUCTION

The parapharyngeal space (PPS) is a complex anatomic space lateral to the oropharynx and medial to the mandible. The PPS can generally be conceptualized as an inverted pyramid with the base of the pyramid at the skull base and the apex at the hyoid bone.[1,2] The PPS is typically considered to be bounded medially and

Conflicts: William Ryan is on the scientific advisory boards for Medtronic, Olympus, and Rakuten Medical. Andrew Larson has no declarations of interest.
[a] Department of Otolaryngology—Head and Neck Surgery, Massachusetts Eye and Ear Infirmary, Harvard Medical School, 243 Charles Street, Boston, MA 02114, USA; [b] Division of Head and Neck Oncologic and Endocrine Surgery, Department of Otolaryngology—Head and Neck Surgery, University of California-San Francisco, 1825 4th Street, Fifth Floor, San Francisco, CA 94158, USA
* Corresponding author.
E-mail address: Andrew_Larson@meei.harvard.edu

anteriorly by the buccopharyngeal fascia surrounding the superior constrictor muscle, laterally by the medial pterygoid muscle, and posteriorly by the prevertebral fascia. The space is divided by the stylohyoid ligament into prestyloid and poststyloid compartments. The prestyloid compartment consists of fat, lymph nodes, and the deep medial extent of the deep lobe of the parotid gland. The poststyloid compartment contains neurovascular structures, including the internal jugular vein, internal carotid artery, and cranial nerves IX, X, XI, and XII.[3]

Although the traditional approach to PPS masses has been transcervical, the transoral approach to the PPS was described as early as 1963 by McIlrath and ReMine.[4] It was not until the 1980s that in a series of cases a range of pathologic conditions were reported to be safely removed via an open transoral approach.[5,6]

With the expansion of intraoperative technology, including rigid endoscopy, and, in particular, transoral robotic surgery (TORS), transoral approaches to PPS masses have been enhanced with the improved visualization and tissue manipulation. Although most tumors removed via a transoral approach are benign and salivary in origin, most commonly pleomorphic adenoma, multiple tumor types have been removed according to published reports (**Box 1** provides a full list).[2,7–14]

In this review article, the authors highlight indications for transoral removal of PPS masses, delineate techniques for the transoral approach to the PPS with an emphasis the on the TORS method of dissection, underline limitations to the transoral approaches, and summarize the outcomes and complications data currently available for tumors removed transorally.

INDICATIONS FOR THE TRANSORAL APPROACH

Before the advent of endoscopic-assisted and TORS approaches, many surgeons considered only small lesions that project into the oropharynx without poststyloid extension to be amenable to open transoral excision.[15,16] Safety concerns of the open transoral approach with limited exposure and poor visualization of key structures included major vascular injury, tumor spillage/capsule violation, incomplete tumor excision, and a presumed possibility of infection with exposure to intraoral microbiome.[11,16–19]

Box 1
Parapharyngeal pathologic condition reported to be removed via transoral approach in existing literature

Pathologic condition

Benign salivary neoplasm (most commonly pleomorphic adenoma)

Hemangioma

Lipoma

Lymphoepithelial cyst/benign cyst

Schwannoma

Parathyroid adenoma

Venous malformation

Malignant salivary neoplasm

Metastatic thyroid carcinoma

The indications for transoral excision of PPS masses have expanded with TORS and transoral endoscopy. Larger, well-circumscribed tumors even with poststyloid involvement can be removed transorally with an acceptable safety profile.[20] Tumors up to 8 cm in diameter have been reported to be successfully removed solely via a transoral TORS approach.[2] Important factors to consider preoperatively include any trismus, which may limit the intraoral exposure and prohibit proper placement of robotic instruments, and the relationship of the tumor to the carotid artery. Tumors that displace the carotid laterally are amenable to transoral excision; however, if the tumor appears infiltrative radiographically, has a poorly defined plane with the great vessels, or displaces the carotid medially, a transcervical approach should be considered.[21]

In addition, if the surgeon is contemplating a solely transoral approach to a PPS mass, the superior and lateral extent of the tumor must be carefully considered. Even when the TORS system is used, lateral extension of the tumor through the stylomandibular tunnel may require a transcervical assist approach through an ipsilateral neck incision that can be less than 4 cm.[20,22] Accordingly, if there is concern for lateral extension of the tumor radiographically during the preoperative consultation, consenting the patient for possible transcervical approach is advised. Furthermore, extension of the tumor toward the skull base may create difficulties with visualization and dissection of the superior portion of the tumor transorally, possibly leading to tumor capsule disruption. Boyce and colleagues[20] suggested that tumors greater than 10 mm from the skull base radiographically are appropriate for TORS excision. A combined transoral-transcervical approach, or an even altogether different skull base approach, should be used to safely access tumors closer than 1 cm to the base of skull.

ADVANTAGES AND DISADVANTAGES OF THE TRANSORAL APPROACH

The main advantages of pursuing a transoral approach to a PPS mass include lack of an external neck scar, avoidance of neck numbness, and near elimination of the possibility of first bite syndrome. A transoral approach also diminishes the risks of facial nerve (in particular, the marginal mandibular branch of the facial nerve) and hypoglossal nerve injury, although the glossopharyngeal nerve is at greater risk during a transoral dissection. In addition, the transoral approach also avoids the risk of Frey syndrome and sialocele from transparotid salivary tissue dissection.[1,17,18,23]

There are drawbacks to the transoral approach. The main drawback of transoral approaches is the more limited exposure. The narrow corridor of dissection can present challenges to dissecting around the full tumor and to controlling bleeding. However, rapid conversion to an open transcervical approach for control of bleeding with vessel ligation is an option. The transoral approach does involve an incision through the superior constrictor and soft palate muscles and dissection through the parapharyngeal fat where vagal nerve branch contributions to the palate and superior constrictor muscles may be affected by interruption or traction injury. Despite these anatomic and surgical factors, patients typically initiate a diet on the first day after surgery.[8] However, longer-term functional and/or quality-of-life (QOL) data comparing swallowing outcomes between transcervical and transoral approaches are not available to fully understand the consequences of the transoral incision and dissection. Bimanual palpation is not possible via a transoral approach. The TORS dissection specifically lacks haptic feedback from the robotic instruments, which may lead to higher rates of tumor capsule disruption. For this reason, one can interrupt the robotic dissection to perform blunt finger dissection of the tumor transorally to digitally gauge the tumor and gently dissect the tumor from surrounding fascial attachments.[15] Pressure on the skin overlying the parotid can result in a push of the parapharyngeal tissue medially that can in turn improve angles of dissection.

The tight corridor for dissection can also challenge a surgeon not facile with endoscopic or robotic dissection. There is a learning curve for a head and neck surgeon to develop these techniques. TORS offers the 3-dimensional optical magnification, a maneuverable endoscope with multiple angles of visualization, and increased degrees of freedom of movement of the robotic arms, all of which can help circumvent the geometric challenges presented by transoral PPS surgery.[24] Ultimately, a simple head light-guided dissection with loupe magnification is an option that can work well for some tumors.

PREOPERATIVE EVALUATION

Careful review of preoperative cross-sectional imaging, typically a computed tomographic (CT) scan or MRI, the latter of which is preferred (**Fig. 1**), is critical to understand the size, location, extent, and presence of infiltration of tumor into surrounding tissues. Cross-sectional imaging should evaluate the skull base, to understand the relationship of the tumor to the skull base, and the full extent of the neck to the clavicles for possible lymphadenopathy. Contrast is helpful to understand the anatomic relationship of the common, internal, and external carotid arteries to the tumor, identify any large feeding vessels, and ensure the appearance of a clear plane between the carotid artery and tumor. Diffusion-weighted MRI additionally can help clarify the malignant potential of salivary tumors preoperatively.[25]

Fine needle aspiration (FNA) is a critical component of the workup of PPS masses. Unless the tumor appears radiologically to be a vascular malformation on MRI, FNA is

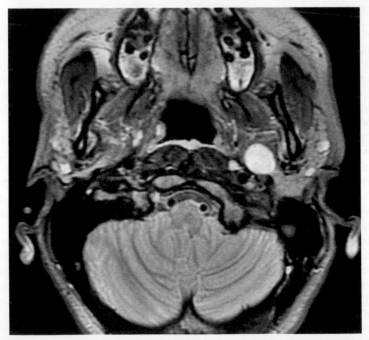

Fig. 1. Sequence of transoral approach to excision of a left PPS acinic cell carcinoma. MRI showing a 2-cm left PPS mass. CT-guided fine needle biopsy showed this to be an acinic cell carcinoma.

recommended for all PPS tumors to clarify the tumor type. In some benign or equivocal tumors, observation with serial imaging of the tumor for growth or changes in imaging characteristics can be a reasonable option; however, an in-depth discussion of the complex decision making surrounding PPS masses is beyond the scope of this article.

The patient's oropharynx should be carefully examined preoperatively to evaluate the following: (1) the extent of tumor visible submucosally; (2) general dental condition for assessing the degree of difficulty with placement of oropharyngeal retractors and if there is a heightened risk for dental damage from loose/decayed teeth; and (3) the presence of trismus, which not only challenges oropharyngeal exposure but also may indicate tumor infiltration into pterygoid musculature. In addition, limited neck mobility, in particular, flexion and extension, can create challenges for the oropharyngeal exposure intraoperatively.

EXPOSURE AND SETUP

Transoral PPS surgery is performed under general anesthesia. Nasotracheal intubation by the anesthesiologist affords maximal exposure of the oropharynx and greater freedom of transoral instruments. Nasotracheal intubation also allows for full closure of the mouth to enable transcervical exposure if needed. The table is turned 180° to allow maximal surgical access around 270° of the head. The neck is extended. The face is protected with a circumferential towel head wrap. The authors typically first attempt exposure with a Crowe-Davis retractor ((Storz, Tuttlingen, Germany) **Fig. 2**). If the soft palate, tonsil, and lateral pharyngeal wall are not well exposed, then exposure with a Feyh-Kastenbauer Weinstein-O'Malley (Olympus Corp., Tokyo, Japan) retractor can be attempted. Generally, retraction of the tongue anteriorly outward with a silk suture passed through the midline tongue is not necessary for the PPS approach. Such retraction can also put the tongue at risk of devascularization from extended compression. If retraction of the tongue with this technique is necessary before engagement of the retractor, the authors recommend regular evaluation of the tongue and intermittent release of the retractor during the course of the operation to allow for tongue revascularization. Facial nerve monitoring should be used for lateral PPS tumors abutting the deep aspect of the parotid to assist with facial nerve identification transorally or if a possible transcervical/transparotid approach is anticipated.

SURGICAL TECHNIQUE: TRANSORAL OPEN APPROACH

In the case whereby a surgical robot or endoscopic instrumentation is not available to a surgeon, or if the surgeon has a greater comfort level with open surgery, an open transoral approach to a PPS tumor may be considered. Loupe magnification and headlight illumination are typically used to improve visualization. Once adequate exposure of the oropharynx has been obtained, an open transoral parapharyngeal dissection may be performed as described by Hussain and colleagues.[2] Palpation of the tumor or transoral ultrasound can be performed before making an incision to guide the extent of incision that is necessary.[12] An incision with monopolar cautery is made lateral to the palatoglossal fold; the incision may be extended superiorly to the soft palate and inferiorly to the base of the tongue and/or floor of mouth as needed to allow safe removal of the mass. A cuff of tissue medial to the gum mucosa is advised to allow for easier suture closure. Dissection through, or lateral to, the palatoglossus muscle will reveal the superior constrictor muscle. An incision made too far laterally and inferiorly will place the lingual nerve at risk of injury. The lingual nerve travels lateral to the medial pterygoid entering this area, and anterior to the medial

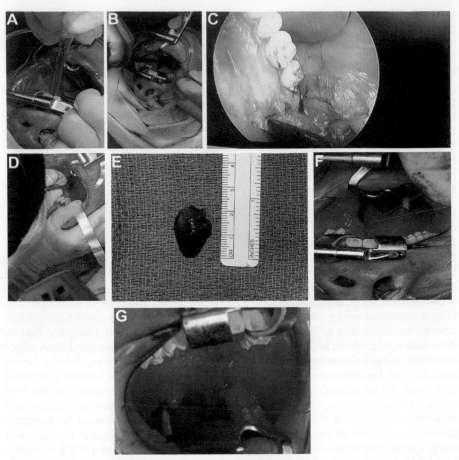

Fig. 2. Sequence of transoral approach to excision of a left PPS acinic cell carcinoma. (*A*) Oral exposure with incision in the left lateral palate and medial retromolar trigone area. (*B*) Incision through the superior constrictor muscle with medial retraction of the tonsil, palate mucosa, superior constructor, and palate musculature for access to the PPS. (*C*) Endoscopic video of the tumor in the PPS after initial medial dissection. (*D*) Transoral dissection of the tumor with blunt and sharp dissection and unipolar and bipolar electrocautery. (*E*) Tumor excised ex vivo. (*F*) Closure of superior constrictor and soft palate/retromolar trigone mucosa after excision of tumor. (*G*) Full mucosal closure.

pterygoid muscle in the posterior floor of mouth. The superior constrictor muscle and the buccopharyngeal fascia surrounding this should be divided. Elevation of a medial flap consisting of the superior constrictor muscle, tonsil, and palatoglossus and palatopharyngeus muscles will lead to the PPS. Identification of the medial pterygoid muscle, the pterygoid plates, and blood vessels, especially the fascia anteriorly overlying the internal carotid artery posteriorly, can be helpful for orientation. Review of the patient's radiologic scans intraoperatively can be helpful during the initial approach to the tumor if the tumor is small and lateral. Once the capsule of the mass has been encountered, careful blunt dissection around the tumor capsule should be performed to release surrounding fascial attachments. If possible, leaving an area of fat and fascia on the capsule of at least part of the tumor can be helpful to be able to manipulate the tumor in different directions without causing an iatrogenic capsule violation. Blunt dissection can be performed at times with gentle finger dissection, the advantage of which is the sensory feedback and ability to adjust pressure. Division of the stylomandibular ligament may facilitate dissection and tumor removal if possible, although this maneuver transorally may be difficult. Once the tumor is removed en bloc, meticulous hemostasis should be achieved. The incision can be closed in 2 layers, with closure of the deeper superior constrictor and palate musculature in a simple interrupted manner and then the mucosa in a horizontal mattress manner with absorbable suture (typically, 3-0 Vicryl suture is used in the authors' practice). A 1-cm area of the inferior portion of the incision can be left open to allow gravity-dependent egress of fluid from the wound. A sequence of this technique is shown in **Fig. 2**.

SURGICAL TECHNIQUE: TRANSORAL ROBOTIC SURGERY APPROACH

When feasible, utilization of a TORS system for transoral removal of a PPS tumor is an option. After exposure of the oropharynx, with insertion of the surgical robot into the operating field, the authors recommend the dissector be placed in the surgical arm contralateral to the tumor and the monopolar cautery be placed on the ipsilateral side. A 0° robotic scope will often give adequate visualization for a PPS tumor; however, a beveled 30° can be used to visualize around more acute angles.

For a TORS transoral approach to the PPS, the dissection is performed similarly to the approach described above, but with some notable exceptions.[15,26] Again, an incision is made near the pterygomandibular raphe, through the palatoglossus and superior constrictor muscles into the PPS while avoiding the lingual nerve. Any tonsillar branches of the external carotid artery system encountered should be ligated with surgical clips deployed by an assistant at the head of the bed. Once the tumor is encountered, careful blunt dissection should be performed around the tumor capsule. Blunt dissection can be facilitated by finger or hand instrument dissection to remove surrounding fascial attachments, which necessarily involves removal of the robotic arms and endoscope from the oropharynx. Although this process of removing and replacing the robotic arms can be time-consuming, the safety and effectiveness of finger and possible hand instrument dissection, with the decreased risk of tumor capsule violation, make this maneuver a worthwhile addition to the operation. Once all fascial and muscular attachments have been released, the tumor is delivered through the incision transorally by the assistant. Again, having a handle of tissue to be able to grasp and move the tumor is helpful, if possible.

The tumor capsule should be carefully inspected for any evidence of violation or tumor spillage. If these are visualized on inspection of the tumor ex vivo, then the wound should be carefully evaluated for any remaining tumor and copiously irrigated with saline after hemostasis has been achieved. After the robotic arms and scope have been removed, the incision is closed in a similar fashion with surgical loupes and headlight as described above for the transoral open approach.

SURGICAL TECHNIQUE: ENDOSCOPE-ASSISTED TRANSORAL APPROACH

The endoscope-assisted transoral technique is similar to the transoral open approach described above, but with extra visualization provided by 0°, 30°, and 45° 5-mm endoscopes (see **Fig. 2**, part C). An assistant can help by holding the endoscope along with a retractor or suction, to allow for adequate multiple-instrument surgery. This technique can be a helpful adjunct to assist removal of these tumors. Numerous investigators facile in endoscopic surgery have reported a good experience with this technique for transoral removal of PPS tumors.[27–32]

SURGICAL TECHNIQUE: TRANSCERVICAL ASSIST TO THE TRANSORAL APPROACH

When a PPS tumor cannot be adequately mobilized for removal transorally, particularly when a tumor extends laterally through the stylomandibular tunnel, a transcervical approach may be used to facilitate transoral tumor removal, as descried by Boyce and colleagues[20]. To perform this, an ipsilateral horizontal neck incision as small as 2.5 to 4 cm can be made. The platysma is divided, and superior and inferior subplatysmal flaps are elevated. The posterior belly of the digastric muscle is identified, at which point the lateral attachments of the tumor can be dissected free with blunt finger dissection. The stylomandibular ligament may also be released from this approach, which facilitates mobilization of the tumor. Once fully mobile, the tumor can then be delivered transorally. The neck incision is then closed in a multilayer fashion. The authors prefer a closed suction neck drain be placed at the time of neck closure.

POSTOPERATIVE CARE

The patient is extubated in the operating room with admission for observation for 1 to 2 nights before discharge home. Liquid diet the first night and soft diet the next day are appropriate as tolerated by the patient. The patient is seen for a follow-up visit in clinic within 1 week postoperatively, at which time the diet can be advanced to a regular diet provided that healing is deemed to be adequate.

TRANSORAL PARAPHARYNGEAL SPACE DISSECTION: COMPLICATIONS AND OUTCOMES

Complications, although unlikely, include unanticipated cranial nerve deficits, including the sympathetic chain, major vascular injury, trismus, and oral mucosal incision dehiscence.[8,15] One report exists of CN X dysfunction following combined transoral-transcervical removal of a large neurogenic tumor, which was dissected free from the vagus nerve, but there are no reports, to the authors' knowledge, of cranial nerve deficits following a purely transoral approach to a PPS tumor.[22] Likewise, major intraoperative vascular injury during the transoral dissection requiring intervention by an interventional radiologist or vascular surgeon has not been reported in existing literature. Two reports of dehiscence of the pharyngeal incision following a TORS approach to PPS tumors highlight that this development can be managed conservatively with a nasogastric feeding tube and oral diet restriction until secondary healing has ensued, as both patients were treated successfully in this manner without further sequelae.[15]

One of the most frequent criticisms of the transoral approach to PPS tumors, in particular pleomorphic adenomas, is higher possible rates of tumor capsule disruption relative to transcervical approaches. Capsule disruption or tumor spillage during the dissection has been shown to be associated with higher rates of tumor recurrence.[33] Capsular disruption rates of pleomorphic adenomas of the PPS during TORS dissection have been reported to be as high as 27%, higher than those reported with transcervical approaches.[20,34] This may be at least partially due to the lack of haptic feedback during a robotic dissection, underscoring the importance of blunt transoral finger dissection during a TORS approach to these tumors.

Recurrent pleomorphic adenomas are not usually detected until, on average, around 10 years following initial resection.[35] As such, there are not yet enough long-term outcomes data from tumors removed via the relatively modern TORS or any oral approach to understand whether recurrence rates are different among PPS tumors removed with TORS, conventional transoral approaches, or more traditional transcervical approaches. Recurrences of tumors in the PPS can be challenging to re-resect and are more morbid, requiring possible pharyngeal resection, mandibulotomy/mandibulectomy, and possible free-flap reconstruction.[23,36]

Validated QOL data and objective functional outcomes data on speech, and in particular swallowing, are not yet published for patients having undergone transoral approaches to removal of PPS tumors. Such data could better illuminate the longer-term subjective outcomes of patients undergoing such procedures.

SUMMARY

Transoral excision of PPS tumors has expanded given the improvements in endo-scopic and robotic surgical technology and comfort with transoral approaches in gen-eral. Even some large tumors with poststyloid extension can be removed safely via a transoral approach. When the lateral aspect of the tumor cannot be adequately mobi-lized transorally, a transcervical assist incision may be used to facilitate transoral tu-mor removal. Longer-term outcomes data will be necessary to delineate whether transoral excision of PPS tumors leads to differing recurrence rates of tumors and QOL/functional outcomes compared with those removed by traditional transcervical approaches. Care must be taken to avoid tumor spillage. Use of transoral, transcervi-cal, or both approaches should be considered to enable the safest and most effective resection.

REFERENCES

1. Carrau RL, Myers EN, Johnson JT. Management of tumors arising in the para-pharyngeal space. Laryngoscope 1990;100(6):583–9.
2. Hussain A, Ah-See KW, Shakeel M. Trans-oral resection of large parapharyngeal space tumours. Eur Arch Otorhinolaryngol 2013;271(3):575–82.
3. Som PM, Curtin HD. Lesions of the parapharyngeal space. Role of MR imaging. Otolaryngol Clin North Am 1995;28(3):515–42.
4. McIlrath DC, ReMine WH. Parapharyngeal tumors. Surg Clin North Am 1963; 43(4):1014–20.
5. Som PM, Biller HF, Lawson W. Tumors of the parapharyngeal space preoperative evaluation, diagnosis and surgical approaches. Ann Otol Rhinol Laryngol 1981; 90(1_suppl3):3–15.
6. Goodwin WJ, Chandler JR. Transoral excision of lateral parapharyngeal space tu-mors presenting intraorally. Laryngoscope 1988;98(3):266–9.
7. Kane AC, Walvekar RR, Hotaling JM. Transoral robotic resection of a retrophar-yngeal parathyroid adenoma: a case report. J Robotic Surg 2018;13(2):335–8.
8. Chan JYK, Tsang RK, Eisele DW, et al. Transoral robotic surgery of the paraphar-yngeal space: a case series and systematic review. Head Neck 2015;37(2): 293–8.
9. Granell J, Alonso A, Garrido L, et al. Transoral fully robotic dissection of a para-pharyngeal hemangioma. J Craniofac Surg 2010;27(7):1806–7.
10. Lajud SA, Aponte-Ortiz JA, Garraton M, et al. A novel combined transoral and transcervical surgical approach for recurrent metastatic medullary thyroid cancer to the parapharyngeal space. J Robotic Surg 2019;14(1):233–6.
11. Kuet M-L, Kasbekar AV, Masterson L, et al. Management of tumors arising from the parapharyngeal space: a systematic review of 1,293 cases reported over 25 years. Laryngoscope 2014;125(6):1372–81.
12. Goepfert RP, Liu C, Ryan WR. Trans-oral robotic surgery and surgeon-performed trans-oral ultrasound for intraoperative location and excision of an isolated

retropharyngeal lymph node metastasis of papillary thyroid carcinoma. Am J Otolaryng 2015;36(5):710–4.

13. Andrews GA, Kwon M, Clayman G, et al. Technical refinement of ultrasound-guided transoral resection of parapharyngeal/retropharyngeal thyroid carcinoma metastases. Head Neck 2011;33(2):166–70.

14. Le TD, Cohen JI. Transoral approach to removal of the retropharyngeal lymph nodes in well-differentiated thyroid cancer. Laryngoscope 2007;117(7):1155–8.

15. O'Malley BW, Quon H, Leonhardt FD, et al. Robotic surgery for parapharyngeal space tumors. Orl 2010;72(6):332–6.

16. Riffat F, Dwivedi RC, Palme C, et al. A systematic review of 1143 parapharyngeal space tumors reported over 20 years. Oral Oncol 2014;50(5):421–30.

17. Dimitrijevic MV, Jesic SD, Mikic AA, et al. Parapharyngeal space tumors: 61 case reviews. Int J Oral Maxillofac Surg 2010;39(10):983–9.

18. Pang KP, Goh CHK, Tan HM. Parapharyngeal space tumours: an 18 year review. J Laryngol Otol 2002;116(3):170–5.

19. Zhi K, Ren W, Zhou H, et al. Management of parapharyngeal-space tumors. J Oral Maxillofac Surg 2009;67(6):1239–44.

20. Boyce BJ, Curry JM, Luginbuhl A, et al. Transoral robotic approach to parapharyngeal space tumors: case series and technical limitations. Laryngoscope 2016; 126(8):1776–82.

21. Chu F, Tagliabue M, Giugliano G, et al. From transmandibular to transoral robotic approach for parapharyngeal space tumors. Am J Otolaryng 2017;38(4):375–9.

22. Betka J, Chovanec M, Klozar J, et al. Transoral and combined transoral–transcervical approach in the surgery of parapharyngeal tumors. Eur Arch Otorhinol 2010;267(5):765–72.

23. Khafif A, Segev Y, Kaplan DM, et al. Surgical management of parapharyngeal space tumors: a 10-year review. Otolaryngol Head Neck Surg 2005;132(3): 401–6.

24. Chan JYK, Richmon JD. Transoral robotic surgery (TORS) for benign pharyngeal lesions. Otolaryngol Clin North Am 2014;47(3):407–13.

25. Yabuuchi H, Matsuo Y, Kamitani T, et al. Parotid gland tumors: can addition of diffusion-weighted MR imaging to dynamic contrast-enhanced MR imaging improve diagnostic accuracy in characterization? Radiology 2008;249(3):909–16.

26. Rassekh CH, Weinstein GS, Loevner LA, et al. Transoral robotic surgery for pre-styloid parapharyngeal space masses. Oper Tech Otolaryngol 2013;24(2): 99–105.

27. Meng L, Zhong Q, Fang J, et al. Early experience in endoscopic transoral resection for parapharyngeal space tumors. Ear Nose Throat J 2018;97(4–5):E5–9.

28. Yaslikaya S, Koca CF, Toplu Y, et al. Endoscopic transoral resection of parapharyngeal osteoma: a case report. J Oral Maxillofac Surg 2016;74(11):2329.e1–5.

29. Sun X, Yan B, Truong H, et al. A comparative analysis of endoscopic-assisted transoral and transnasal approaches to parapharyngeal space: a cadaveric study. J Neurol Surg B Skull Base 2017;79(03):229–40.

30. Li S-Y, Hsu C-H, Chen M-K. Minimally invasive endoscope-assisted trans-oral excision of huge parapharyngeal space tumors. Auris Nasus Larynx 2015; 42(2):179–82.

31. Liu Y, Yu H-J, Zhen H-T. Transoral and endoscope-assisted transoral approaches to resecting benign tumours of the parapharyngeal space located in the medial portion of the carotid sheaths and extending toward the skull base: our experience. J Laryngol Otol 2018;132(8):748–52.

32. Iseri M, Ozturk M, Kara A, et al. Endoscope-assisted transoral approach to parapharyngeal space tumors. Head Neck 2015;37(2):243–8.
33. Witt RL. The significance of the margin in parotid surgery for pleomorphic adenoma. Laryngoscope 2002;112(12):2141–54.
34. Hughes KV, Olsen KD, McCaffrey TV. Parapharyngeal space neoplasms. Head Neck 1995;17(2):124–30.
35. Henriksson G, Westrin KM, Carlson B, et al. Recurrent primary pleomorphic adenomas of salivary gland origin: intrasurgical rupture, histopathologic features, and pseudopodia. Cancer 1998;82(4):617–20.
36. Cassoni A, Terenzi V, Monaca MD, et al. Parapharyngeal space benign tumours: our experience. J Craniomaxillofac Surg 2013;42(2):101–5.

Management of Mucoceles, Sialoceles, and Ranulas

Eve M.R. Bowers, BA[a], Barry Schaitkin, MD[b],*

KEYWORDS

- Mucocele • Ranula • Sialocele • Lip • Mouth floor • Marsupialization
- Surgical management

KEY POINTS

- Mucoceles are benign, mucin-filled cysts commonly found on the bottom lip, and are frequently managed with surgical excision.
- Sialoceles are a variant of mucocele that develop from the extravasation of saliva from injured parotid parenchyma. Acute salivary ductal injuries should be repaired when possible. Delayed presentations may require botulinum toxin or surgery for resolution.
- Ranulas are a type of mucocele that can vary from superficial floor-of-mouth lesions to plunging neck masses. Ranulas are extravasation pseudocysts that are most commonly managed by surgical excision of the cyst and the associated sublingual gland.

INTRODUCTION

Mucoceles, sialoceles, and ranulas are extravasation pseudocysts. The collection of mucus itself does not have an epithelial lining; therefore, removing the pseudocyst generally does not solve the problem. Each of these entities is discussed in turn for their unique aspects. The most common treatment modalities are highlighted.

Mucocele

Mucoceles are common, oral lesions that most frequently present as painless, clear or bluish cysts on the bottom lip of young adults and children. They are benign, mucus-filled growths that typically occur from damage to minor salivary glands or ducts **(Fig. 1)**. Injury to the salivary glands through lip biting, sucking, or trauma can cause mucus to leak into surrounding subepithelial tissue, resulting in the most common variant of mucocele called a mucus extravasation cyst.[1] Mucoceles may also develop from mucus buildup behind blocked glandular ducts, resulting in a less common

Conflicts of interest: None.
[a] Department of Otolaryngology, University of Pittsburgh Medical Center, University of Pittsburgh School of Medicine, 3550 Terrace Street, Pittsburgh, PA 15213, USA; [b] Department of Otolaryngology, University of Pittsburgh Medical Center, Shadyside Hospital, Suite 211, 5200 Centre Avenue, Pittsburgh, PA 15232, USA
* Corresponding author.
E-mail address: schaitkinb@upmc.edu

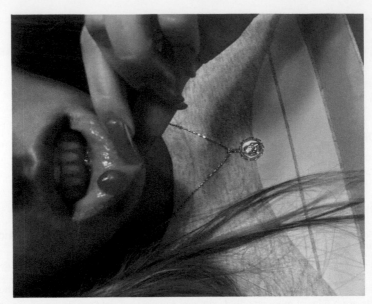

Fig. 1. Patient with lower lip mucocele.

variant of mucocele called a mucus retention cyst.[2] This type of mucocele is most common in individuals between 50 and 60 years old and is typically located in the cheek or palate. On histology, retention cysts have an epithelial lining, whereas extravasation cysts do not.[1,3]

Sixty-six percent of all mucoceles present in patients less than 30 years old, with a peak incidence in the second decade of life and no predilection for gender. The most common location is the lower labial mucosa, with up to 80% of all mucoceles occurring on either side of the lower lip.[4,5] The prevalence of all oral mucoceles is 2.5 in 1000. The size does not usually exceed 10 mm in diameter.[6,7] Two case studies of oral mucoceles reported that almost all included lip mucoceles were histologically characteristic of extravasation cysts, which corroborates the hypothesis that lip mucoceles are commonly incited by traumatic injury such as tooth impingement.[6,8] Although frequently asymptomatic, mucoceles may interfere with chewing, eating, and speech, and may be cosmetically unappealing.[9] Common differential diagnoses for these lesions include oral hemangioma, fibroma, soft tissue abscess, oral lymphangioma, salivary duct cyst, epidermoid cyst, and lipoma.[10] Lip mucoceles are diagnosed clinically based on pathognomonic appearance, location, history of trauma, time to manifestation, cyst hue, and texture. Palpation for mobility and fluctuance helps narrow the differential diagnosis in many cases.[6]

Although oral mucoceles may resolve without treatment, recurrence is common. Additional interventions may be required to remove enlarged cysts or to prevent relapse. Although lacrimal catheters can be used to recannulate a blocked glandular duct in the case of retention cysts,[10] retention and extravasation mucocele cysts are generally both best excised. Conventional surgical excision with removal of surrounding small salivary ducts remains the most common treatment of small mucoceles because of low recurrence, with 1 case series showing a recurrence rate of 4.3% 3 years following complete surgical excision.[5,11] Large mucoceles may be removed surgically using marsupialization to avoid damaging surrounding structures, particularly the labial branch of the mental nerve.[12,13] Marsupialization involves unroofing the mucocele through a small intralesional mucosal incision to remove the mucinous material. Recurrence can be prevented by excising the minor salivary gland before performing primary closure.[5,14] Micromarsupialization is a minimally invasive procedure that involves tying a surgical knot with silk suture at the widest diameter of the mucocele. The mucocele should recede by time of suture removal 7 to 10 days after placement. Recurrences occur 14.2% of the time; however, the series was based on a small number of patients. The procedure is fast and relatively painless, making it a popular option for pediatric patients.[15]

Although surgical removal is common, lip disfigurement, damage to adjacent ducts, numbness, and scarring are complications; thus, some investigators propose a first-line treatment alternative with CO_2 laser ablation.[5,10,16,17] CO_2 laser ablation is a fast and simple technique limited to the superficial mucosa when set between 5 and 10 W. CO_2 laser ablation has limited postoperative bleeding, pain, complications, and damage to surrounding structures, and shorter healing time and relapse, compared with scalpel excision.[5,16–18] Because it does not require suture, CO_2 laser ablation typically takes 3 to 5 minutes. The bloodless nature of the procedure allows excellent surgical visibility.[19]

Cryotherapy and intralesional steroid injection have also been introduced as first-line treatments but are associated with high rates of lesion recurrence, often requiring surgical reintervention.[20,21] Cryotherapy uses the application of extreme cold via cryogen agents such as nitrous oxide or liquid nitrogen to destroy mucoceles during alternating freeze-thaw cycles. It is painless, quick, and simple. The drawbacks include that it can require multiple applications and has limited use for deep lesions.[21–23]

The sclerosing agents OK-432 (picibanil) and polidocanol are less commonly used but have been reported to be effective in curing mucoceles by sealing the traumatized mucinous gland capsule through collapse of the cyst wall.[24–26] Although OK-432 has been associated with shock, fever, and a recurrence rate of 14.3%, a recent study using polidocanol reported a cure rate of 91% with no significant side effects.[27,28]

Although there is no unanimous consensus on the best management of mucoceles, surgical excision is low cost, highly effective, and commonly used. CO_2 laser may represent an effective alternative to surgical excision because of the benefits of minimal postoperative discomfort and good wound healing.[26]

Sialocele

Traumatic sialoceles are common complications of iatrogenic parotid duct injury, neoplasm, infection, trauma, or stenosis of the duct with subsequent duct expansion.[29] These saliva-containing, subcutaneous clefts are a variation of mucocele that form through the extravasation of saliva from injured parotid tissue into the surrounding periglandular space (**Fig. 2**). The duct remains intact in some cases.[30] Superficial lesions present as soft and mobile swellings on the side of the injury, whereas deeper cysts may be difficult to palpate because of overlying tissues. Sialoceles typically present 8 to 14 days after parotid duct trauma. They are painless unless infected, in which case they may transform into external salivary fistulae.[30] Fine-needle aspiration shows high salivary amylase concentration, typically more than 10,000 U/L. Sialography or MRI may be useful at times for diagnosis.[30,31,33]

Surgeons most commonly encounter sialoceles after parotidectomy. Essentially all parotid surgeries, superficial or total, leave residual parotid salivary tissue behind. In the immediate postoperative period, patients frequently leak saliva into the soft tissues. Initial conservative management of traumatic sialoceles is preferred, especially in small and superficial duct injuries. Treatment of these collections has included pressure dressings, aspiration, delayed suction drains, medications to

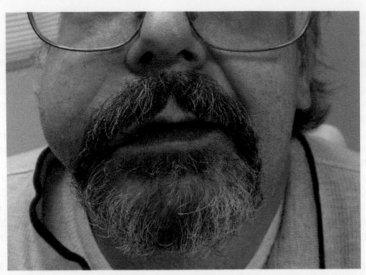

Fig. 2. Chronic right parotid sialocele after windshield laceration to the face and failure to identify and repair the ductal injury acutely. Botox injections successfully treated this lesion.

decrease saliva production, radiation, and botulinum toxin. Propantheline-bromide is an anticholinergic antisialogogue frequently used to inhibit parotid secretion through the healing phase, although unwanted anticholinergic side effects require monitoring.[32,34,35] Although aspiration with compression is common, Witt[36] showed that there is no difference in the results of aspirating versus not aspirating postoperative sialoceles. Radiation therapy can result in fibrosis and gland degeneration but should be avoided if possible. Because sialoceles almost all go away while being ignored, only large and very persistent ones need to be treated with botulinum toxin. There are few articles with information on doing this. A recent review article found 47 total cases reported. There is currently no agreed-on dose for the treatment of sialoceles and, in this article, doses ranged from 45 to 200 units. The botulinum toxin is injected into the remaining salivary gland tissue after aspirating the pseudocyst. It has been described with or without ultrasonography guidance. Additional collection of saliva may occur for a short time after chemodenervation. Success rates range from 70% to 100%.[37] In general, time is the best treatment of most of these postsurgical problems.

Parotid duct injuries otherwise causing sialoceles are penetrating lacerations most commonly from an assault weapon, knife, or glass shard.[38] Ideally, these are managed acutely with immediate identification of the proximal and distal ends and repairing them either primarily or with a vein interposition graft to redirect parotid secretions into the mouth. Failure to reconstitute the duct risks sialocele formation and cutaneous fistula. The presence of a foreign body should be considered if a traumatic sialocele develops (**Fig. 3**). Parotid duct reconstruction can be complicated by difficulty locating the proximal end of the duct caused by scarring, and facial nerve damage while attempting this procedure has been reported.[39,40] There is no publication detailing the long-term patency rate of reconstituted parotid ducts. Conventional or magnetic resonance sialography or ultrasonography can help to identify a complete obstruction of the duct. Recannulation of the parotid duct using salivary endoscopy is challenging. However, proximal sialoceles have been successfully connected to normal distal ducts with salivary endoscopic assistance and stenting.[41]

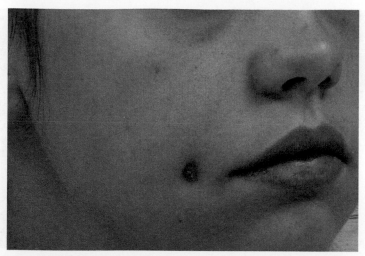

Fig. 3. Chronic right parotid sialocele and fistula that resolved with identifying and removing foreign body, which in this case was a remnant of the original penetrating stick.

Case reports describe tympanic neurectomy as a denervation alternative for salivary fistula and sialocele. Sectioning of the auriculotemporal or Jacobsen nerve prevents parotid gland secretion by inhibiting parasympathetic supply to the gland; however, there is a large risk of failure or recurrence. Botulinum toxin acts by inhibiting acetylcholine release, which inhibits secretomotor parasympathetic nerve activity, causing decreased saliva production.[42] It has been used safely and effectively in small case series.[29,32] Some failures after initial improvement have been reported. If the duct continuity cannot be reestablished, and botulinum toxin is only successful for the 3 months following injection, then surgical glandular extirpation may be required.

Ranula

Ranulas are a subset of mucocele that present on the floor of the mouth as painless, fluctuant, blue-hued, mobile masses.[43] Ranulas are classified as either simple or plunging. Simple ranula pseudocysts, limited to the submucosa of the floor of mouth, typically arise from trauma to the sublingual glands (although there may be no history of such). Plunging ranulas are defined by the penetration of mucocele content through fascial planes, often posterior to or through the mylohyoid muscle (**Fig. 4**).[44] These lesions can extend superiorly, posteriorly, or inferiorly into the parapharyngeal, retropharyngeal, and supraclavicular/superior mediastinal areas respectively and may present as cervical masses.[27,44,45] Sometimes plunging ranulas exist without a visible floor-of-mouth component.

The incidence of ranulas is 0.2 in 1000, arising from the sublingual gland more than 90% of the time.[14] Like lip mucoceles, the diagnosis is typically based on history and clinical picture, although imaging modalities and biopsy can be used. Fine-needle aspiration cytology findings of a high amylase content, histiocytes, and no epithelial cells is helpful in differentiating ranulas from other oral or neck masses such as thyroglossal duct cyst, branchial cleft cyst, cystic hygroma/lymphatic malformation, intramuscular hemangioma, lymphangioma, abscess, or dermoid.[45]

Ranulas are surgically removed an estimated 80% of the time. The management is similar to that of lip mucoceles with some variation. Superficial and plunging ranulas should be treated with surgical removal of the ranula and implicated sublingual gland

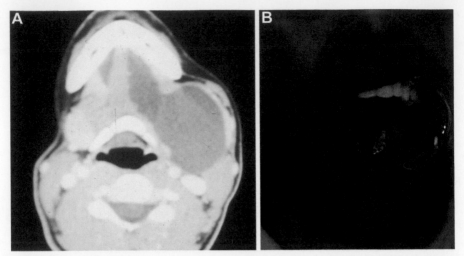

Fig. 4. (*A*) Computed tomography scan of left-sided plunging ranula. (*B*) Clinical view of large left ranula. Plunging neck mass can be seen in left submandibular triangle.

via a transoral approach. Sublingual gland excision is preferred to marsupialization because of much lower rates of ranula recurrence.[14,46–50] A transcervical approach with neck exploration for plunging ranulas is not necessary. Plunging ranulas can be effectively treated by removing the sublingual gland transorally and evacuating the extravasated mucus through the transoral approach.[51,52] Ranulas almost never recur when the sublingual gland is excised; however, avoiding injury to the adjacent submandibular duct or lingual nerve during excision is important.[27,53–56] Recurrence rates of superficial ranulas removed with excision without the associated gland is reported to be between 25% and 56.69%. Ranulas treated by marsupialization recur at rates between 36.4% and 66.7%.[54]

Kono and colleagues[57] conducted a retrospective chart review including 23 patients with intraoral ranulas treated with OK-432 (picibanil) injection sclerosing therapy. The overall efficacy rate was 91.2% without complications. Complete regression of intraoral ranulas occurred in 78.2% of patients. More than 1 injection is required in most patients for complete cure. The drug is more effective in small lesions.[57]

SUMMARY

Mucoceles are benign extravasation pseudocysts. Lip mucoceles, sialoceles, and ranulas are variations of mucoceles that can be managed medically or surgically depending on the type. Lip mucoceles are generally treated with surgery, whereas sialoceles should be managed conservatively or with botulinum toxin or surgery in delayed presentations. Ranulas are managed with surgical removal of the cyst wall and associated sublingual gland and evacuation of the pseudocyst.

CLINICS CARE POINTS

(1) Ideal treatment of salivary collections is determined by the presence or absence of a true epithelial lining.

(2) The presence of a true cyst lining makes marsupialization possible.

(3) Both true cysts and pseudocysts can recur if the source generator persists.

AUTHOR CONTRIBUTIONS

Concept and design: E.M.R. Bowers, B. Schaitkin.
Analysis and interpretation: E.M.R. Bowers, B. Schaitkin.
Data collection: E.M.R. Bowers, B. Schaitkin.
Writing the article: E.M.R. Bowers, B. Schaitkin.
Critical revision of the article: E.M.R. Bowers, B. Schaitkin.
Final approval of the article: B. Schaitkin.
Statistical analysis: not relevant.
Obtain funding: none obtained.
Overall responsibility: B. Schaitkin.

REFERENCES

1. Senthilkumar B, Mahabob MN. Mucocele: An unusual presentation of the minor salivary gland lesion. J Pharm Bioallied Sci 2012;4(Suppl 2):S180–2.
2. Boneu Bonet F, Vidal Homs E, Maizcurrana Tornil A, et al. Mucocele de la glandula submaxilar: a propósito de un caso. Med Oral Patol Oral Cir Bucal 2005; 10:180–4.
3. Bodner L, Tal H. Salivary gland cysts of the oral cavity: clinical observation and surgical management. Compendium 1991;12(3):154–6, 150, 152.
4. Silva A Jr, Nikitakis NG, Balciunas BA, et al. Superficial mucocele of the labial mucosa: a case report and review of the literature. Gen Dent 2004;52(5):424–7.
5. Yague-Garcia J, Espana-Tost AJ, Berini-Aytes L, et al. Treatment of oral mucocele-scalpel versus CO2 laser. Med Oral Patol Oral Cir Bucal 2009;14(9): e469–74.
6. Yamasoba T, Tayama N, Syoji M, et al. Clinicostatistical study of lower lip mucoceles. Head Neck 1990;12(4):316–20.
7. Bouquot JE, Gundlach KK. Oral exophytic lesions in 23,616 white Americans over 35 years of age. Oral Surg Oral Med Oral Pathol 1986;62(3):284–91.
8. Harrison JD. Salivary mucoceles. Oral Surg Oral Med Oral Pathol 1975;39(2): 268–78.
9. Mínguez-Martinez I, Bonet-Coloma C, Ata-Ali-Mahmud J, et al. Clinical characteristics, treatment, and evolution of 89 mucoceles in children. J Oral Maxillofac Surg 2010;68(10):2468–71.
10. Bhargava N, Agarwal P, Sharma N, et al. An unusual presentation of oral mucocele in infant and its review. Case Rep Dent 2014;2014:723130.
11. Bahadure RN, Fulzele P, Thosar N, et al. Conventional surgical treatment of oral mucocele: a series of 23 cases. Eur J Paediatr Dent 2012;13(2):143–6.
12. Ata-Ali J, Carrillo C, Bonet C, et al. Oral mucocele: Review of the literature. J Clin Exp Dentistry 2010;2.
13. Baurmash HD. A case against sublingual gland removal as primary treatment of ranulas. J Oral Maxillofac Surg 2007;65(1):117–21.
14. Baurmash HD. Mucoceles and ranulas. J Oral Maxillofac Surg 2003;61(3): 369–78.
15. Delbem AC, Cunha RF, Vieira AE, et al. Treatment of mucus retention phenomena in children by the micro-marsupialization technique: case reports. Pediatr Dent 2000;22(2):155–8.
16. Huang IY, Chen CM, Kao YH, et al. Treatment of mucocele of the lower lip with carbon dioxide laser. J Oral Maxillofac Surg 2007;65(5):855–8.
17. Niccoli-Filho W, Morosolli AR. Surgical treatment of ranula with carbon dioxide laser radiation. Lasers Med Sci 2004;19(1):12–4.

18. García-Ortiz de Zárate F, España-Tost AJ, Berini-Aytés L, et al. Aplicaciones del láser de CO2 en Odontología. RCOE 2004;9:567–76.

19. Basu MK, Frame JW, Rhys Evans PH. Wound healing following partial glossectomy using the CO2 laser, diathermy and scalpel: a histological study in rats. J Laryngol Otol 1988;102(4):322–7.

20. Sinha R, Sarkar S, Khaitan T, et al. Nonsurgical Management of Oral Mucocele by Intralesional Corticosteroid Therapy. Int J Dent 2016;2016:2896748.

21. Aulakh KK, Brar RS, Azad A, et al. Cryotherapy for Treatment of Mouth Mucocele. Niger J Surg 2016;22(2):130–3.

22. Gill D. Two simple treatments for lower lip mucocoeles. Australas J Dermatol 1996;37(4):220.

23. Garg A, Tripathi A, Chowdhry S, et al. Cryosurgery: painless and fearless management of mucocele in young patient. J Clin Diagn Res 2014;8(8):ZD04–6.

24. Ohta N, Fukase S, Suzuki Y, et al. Treatment of salivary mucocele of the lower lip by OK-432. Auris Nasus Larynx 2011;38(2):240–3.

25. Muraoka M, Taniguchi T, Harada T. A new conservative treatment for retention cyst of the lip: OK-432 injection. Br J Plast Surg 2002;55(6):533.

26. Liu J-L, Zhang A-Q, Jiang L-C, et al. The efficacy of polidocanol sclerotherapy in mucocele of the minor salivary gland. J Oral Pathol Med 2018;47(9):895–9.

27. Arunachalam P, Priyadharshini N. Recurrent plunging ranula. J Indian Assoc Pediatr Surgeons 2010;15(1):36.

28. Re Cecconi D, Achilli A, Tarozzi M, et al. Mucoceles of the oral cavity: a large case series (1994-2008) and a literature review. Med Oral Patol Oral Cir Bucal 2010;15(4):e551–6.

29. Araujo MRd, Centurion BS, Albuquerque DFd, et al. Management of a parotid sialocele in a young patient: case report and literature review. J Appl Oral Sci 2010; 18(4):432–6.

30. Sulabha AN, Sangamesh NC, Warad N, et al. Sialocele: an unusual case report and its management. Indian J Dent Res 2011;22(2):336–9.

31. Canosa A, Cohen MA. Post-traumatic parotid sialocele: Report of two cases. J Oral Maxillofac Surg 1999;57(6):742–5.

32. Parekh D, Glezerson G, Stewart M, et al. Post-traumatic parotid fistulae and sialoceles. A prospective study of conservative management in 51 cases. Ann Surg 1989;209(1):105–11.

33. Langdon JD. Complications of parotid gland surgery. J Maxillofac Surg 1984; 12(5):225–9.

34. Krausen AS, Ogura JH. Sialoceles: medical treatment first. Trans Sect Otolaryngol Am Acad Ophthalmol Otolaryngol 1977;84(5):Orl890–5.

35. Steinberg MJ, Herréra AF. Management of parotid duct injuries. Oral Surg Oral Med Oral Pathol Oral Radiol Endod 2005;99(2):136–41.

36. Witt RL. The incidence and management of siaolocele after parotidectomy. Otolaryngol Head Neck Surg 2009;140(6):871–4.

37. Maharaj S, Mungul S, Laher A. Botulinum toxin A is an effective therapeutic tool for the management of parotid sialocele and fistula: A systematic review. Laryngoscope Investig Otolaryngol 2020;5(1):37–45.

38. Pereira KD, Smith SL, Mitchell RB. Parotid sialocele in a 10-year-old girl. Ear Nose Throat J 2007;86(1):27–8.

39. Demetriades D, Rabinowitz B. Management of parotid sialoceles: a simple surgical technique. Br J Surg 1987;74(4):309.

40. Ananthakrishnan N, Parkash S. Parotid fistulas: a review. Br J Surg 1982;69(11): 641–3.

41. Nahlieli O, Abramson A, Shacham R, et al. Endoscopic treatment of salivary gland injuries due to facial rejuvenation procedures. Laryngoscope 2008; 118(5):763–7.
42. Chow TL, Kwok SP. Use of botulinum toxin type A in a case of persistent parotid sialocele. Hong Kong Med J 2003;9(4):293–4.
43. Packiri S, Gurunathan D, Selvarasu K. Management of paediatric oral ranula: a systematic review. J Clin Diagn Res 2017;11(9):ZE06–9.
44. Davison MJ, Morton RP, McIvor NP. Plunging ranula: clinical observations. Head Neck 1998;20(1):63–8.
45. Sheikhi M, Jalalian F, Rashidipoor R, et al. Plunging ranula of the submandibular area. Dent Res J (Isfahan) 2011;8(Suppl 1):S114–8.
46. Crysdale W, Mendelsohn J, Conley S. Ranulas—mucoceles of the oral cavity: experience in 26 children. Laryngoscope 1988;98(3):296–8.
47. Catone G. Sublingual gland mucus-escape phenomenon treatment by excision of sublingual gland. J Oral Surg 1969;27:774–86.
48. Bridger AG, Carter P, Bridger GP. Plunging ranula: literature review and report of three cases. Aust N Z J Surg 1989;59(12):945–8.
49. O'Connor R, McGurk M. The plunging ranula: diagnostic difficulties and a less invasive approach to treatment. Int J Oral Maxillofac Surg 2013;42(11):1469–74.
50. Kolomvos N, Kalfarentzos E, Papadogeorgakis N. Surgical treatment of plunging ranula: Report of three cases and review of literature. Oral Maxillofac Surg Cases 2019;5:100098.
51. McGurk M. Management of the ranula. J Oral Maxillofac Surg 2007;65(1):115–6.
52. Yoshimura Y, Obara S, Kondoh T, et al. A comparison of three methods used for treatment of ranula. J Oral Maxillofac Surg 1995;53(3):280–2 [discussion: 283].
53. Rho MH, Kim DW, Kwon JS, et al. OK-432 sclerotherapy of plunging ranula in 21 patients: it can be a substitute for surgery. AJNR Am J Neuroradiol 2006;27(5): 1090–5.
54. Choi M-G. Case report of the management of the ranula. J Korean Assoc Oral Maxillofac Surg 2019;45(6):357–63.
55. Mustafa AB, Bokhari K, Luqman M, et al. Plunging ranula: An interesting case report. 2013.
56. Zhao Y-F, Jia J, Jia Y. Complications associated with surgical management of ranulas. J Oral Maxillofac Surg 2005;63(1):51–4.
57. Kono M, Satomi T, Abukawa H, et al. Evaluation of OK-432 Injection Therapy as Possible Primary Treatment of Intraoral Ranula. J Oral Maxillofac Surg 2017;75(2): 336–42.

Transoral Sialolithotomy Without Endoscopes
An Alternative Approach to Salivary Stones

Janyn Quiz, BS, M. Boyd Gillespie, MD, MSc*

KEYWORDS

- Salivary stone • Sialolithiasis • Salivary duct obstruction • Wharton duct
- Submandibular duct • Sialolithotomy • Salivary endoscopy • Sialendoscopy

KEY POINTS

- Most salivary stones cannot be removed with endoscopic techniques alone.
- Most of the salivary stones are amendable to transoral sialolithotomy without use of endoscopes.
- Outcomes of sialolithotomy without endoscopes are comparable to outcomes using scope-based techniques.

 Video content accompanies this article at http://www.oto.theclinics.com.

INTRODUCTION

Sialolithiasis, one of the most common benign pathologies of the major salivary glands, is the formation of stones within the salivary ductal system. Sialoliths are commonly asymptomatic but may present with swelling or pain due to their capacity for ductal obstruction.[1] Evidence suggests that up to 0.45% of the population will experience symptomatic sialolithiasis in their lifetime.[2] There is an estimated overall incidence of 1% to 2% due to spontaneous expulsion of stones that are otherwise asymptomatic. The most commonly reported site of sialolithiasis is the submandibular gland, accounting for more than 80% of the cases, followed by the parotid gland with 10% to 20% and sublingual gland with 1% to 5% of these cases.[3] Little is certain regarding the pathogenesis of sialolithiasis. Prevailing theories assert that a nidus for stone formation results from (1) mucoid salivary proteins precipitated by decreased salivary flow or dehydration; (2) elevated salivary calcium levels that are present; or (3) retrograde flow of bacteria and food into the ductal system.[4,5]

Department of Otolaryngology–Head & Neck Surgery, University of Tennessee Health Science Center, 910 Madison Avenue, Suite 408, Memphis, TN 38163, USA
* Corresponding author.
E-mail address: mgilles8@uthsc.edu

Otolaryngol Clin N Am 54 (2021) 553–565
https://doi.org/10.1016/j.otc.2021.01.006
0030-6665/21/© 2021 Elsevier Inc. All rights reserved.

Imaging is indicated in patients with obstructive salivary disorders in order to determine the likely cause of the obstruction (stone vs nonstone), the number of obstructions (single vs multiple), the features of the obstruction (stone size, shape), and the location of the obstruction (intraglandular, hilum, proximal duct, distal duct, ostium). Historically, radiography was used in the diagnosis of sialolithiasis as an effective way to detect large ductal stones. However, intraglandular, small and radiotransparent ($\sim$20%) stones are easily missed with this modality.[6] Sialography with digital subtraction eventually became the gold standard for diagnosis, as it allows for evaluation of stones and detailed ductal morphology. However, drawbacks include radiation exposure, patient discomfort, and complications such as ductal perforation and infection.[6–8] Currently, the most commonly used noninvasive imaging techniques are ultrasonography and computed tomography (CT). Ultrasound is an excellent imaging choice for obstructive salivary disorders, including stones. Many otolaryngology–head and neck surgery clinics currently have access to ultrasound. Benefits of ultrasound include availability, no radiation exposure, and lower expense compared with other imaging modalities. An additional advantage is the ability to perform a real-time functional examination by administering a sialogogue such as a sour candy before the examination. This will cause a dilation of the obstructed duct, which can then be followed by the ultrasound probe to the pinch point that corresponds to the site of obstruction. Stones will usually appear as hyperechoic lines that reflect the acoustic signal resulting in an area of acoustic shadow behind the stone, and this will allow for measurement of the stone in at least one dimension. In addition, ultrasound can be combined with bimanual examination to improve the visualization of stones that can be palpated intraorally. However, ultrasonography has drawbacks. It is largely operator dependent. Ultrasound is poor at detecting stones measuring less than 2 mm or stones or other ductal pathologies in the anterior floor of mouth. Ultrasound does not generally allow reliable exclusion of sialoliths.[6,8,9] Thin-cut CT scans effectively detect calcifications. However, drawbacks include radiation exposure, relatively high cost to patients, and poor visualization of stenoses and strictures.[3,6] Because of these reasons, CT is reserved for cases in which ultrasonography is not readily available or nondiagnostic. However, CT largely remains the imaging modality of choice in North America due to a higher sensitivity (98%) and specificity (88%) compared with ultrasound, which has a sensitivity of 65% and specificity of 80%.[10]

In 1991, Katz first described sialendoscopy and the application of endoscopic technology to directly visualize ductal morphology and salivary stones.[8,11] Sialendoscopy is highly sensitive and specific with regard to diagnosis, while also allowing for potential therapeutic intervention with stone extraction and stricture dilation. Sialendoscopy has become the gold standard in sialolithiasis treatment, which traditionally involved initial conservative measures (hydration; sialogogues; gland massage; pain control; and antibiotics), followed by salivary gland resection if the obstruction was not relieved. Currently, the goal of sialolithiasis management has transitioned to a gland preservation approach, as studies have shown restoration of normal gland histology and function following relief of obstruction.[12,13] Interventional sialendoscopy techniques have gained the favor of surgeons and patients because these avoid gland extirpation along with the associated side effects of external scar, loss of facial contour, facial numbness, facial weakness, gustatory sweating, and reduced salivary volume.[14]

Because of high effectiveness rates demonstrated by sialendoscopy, it has skyrocketed to the forefront of sialolithiasis evaluation and management. However, this procedure is not without its drawbacks, such as significant costs, patient accessibility with need to travel to a center offering the technique, and complications.[15,16] In addition, certain ductal and sialolith characteristics limit the utility of sialendoscopy.[17] This article aims to discuss the limitations of sialendoscopy, explore the utility of transoral lithotomy, and compare these 2 approaches in order to propose a modified algorithm for sialolithiasis management.

SIALENDOSCOPY AND ITS LIMITATIONS FOR SIALOLITHIASIS

The advent of endoscopic technology aided the goal of gland preservation in the treatment of sialolithiasis. A meta-analysis of 20 studies of sialendoscopy for obstructive salivary diseases demonstrated a pooled success rate, defined as being symptom-free without residual obstruction, of 86% (95% confidence interval [CI], 83% to 89%) for the endoscopy alone and 93% (95% CI, 89% to 96%) when combined with incisional surgical approaches.[18] It is clear that although sialendoscopy is effective, concurrent open approaches are still necessary in many of these cases.

Transoral sialolithotomy is one such surgical approach in which an incision is made within the oral cavity to directly visualize and extract the obstructing calculus. Following stone removal, the duct may or may not be repaired with a formal dochoplasty depending on the level of concern for ongoing obstruction of the distal duct. Although it is commonly used as an adjunct to sialendoscopy, transoral sialolithotomy can stand alone without endoscopy, with reported success rates in the range of 90% to 95%.[19–21] Factors contributing to the success of transoral sialolithotomy are the palpability of the stone and the ability to accurately localize the stone.[21,22] Zenk and colleagues[21] recommend that transoral removal of submandibular duct stones should be the treatment of choice in palpable and/or readily ultrasound-visualized stones due to the high success (94%) and low complication rates (<3%) observed in their patient series. Additional investigators advocate for transoral sialolithotomy having demonstrated that factors such as submandibular duct location, palpability, CT localization, and increased diameter of stones were predictive of an incisional management, independent of sialendoscope availability.[14,23]

At their institution, Juul and Wagner[23] shifted toward transoral sialolithotomy as a standard treatment of larger sialoliths. This strategy was borne from the following reasons: (1) about half of sialendoscopic extraction of stones larger than 7 or 8 mm or irregularly shaped were unsuccessful using sialendoscopy alone; (2) sialendoscopy tended to cause edema of the floor of the oral cavity, which made subsequent adjunctive techniques more difficult to perform; and (3) that there are limited financial resources to maintain scopes that would frequently breakdown after 10 to 20 cases. In their practice, they used imaging characteristics to justify avoiding sialendoscopy for definable large and irregularly shaped stones to reduce risk is sialendoscopy complications such as perforation and scarring. They found a high success rate (93%), high patient satisfaction (94%), a high number of patients without ongoing symptoms (92%), and minimal complications (lingual nerve damage 3% and tingling of the tongue 6%).

In a large series with more than 1000 patients that examined gland-preserving strategies, Zenk and colleagues[24] reported the removal of submandibular sialoliths using transoral sialolithotomy without endoscopes in 92% of cases (n = 681) versus 5% of cases (n = 35) with a purely sialendoscopic approach. Although both procedures enjoyed similar success rates (90% and 93%, respectively), sialendoscopy was often limited by stone size and mobility and the presence of coexisting scar tissue encasing the stone. The mean diameter of stones removed by sialendoscopy was 4.9 mm compared with 9.1 mm for stones removed by transoral sialolithotomy. These results further demonstrate the role for transoral sialolithotomy without endoscopes in certain circumstances.

As with any invasive procedure, both sialendoscopy and transoral sialolithotomy carry the potential for complications. Sialendoscopy-related complications occur in 2% to 3% of cases in experienced hands; however, surgeons who are learning the technique may have complication rates as high as 10%. Common complications include mild sialadenitis, ductal wall perforation, temporary lingual nerve paresthesia, postoperative infection, and traumatic ranula. Incidence of sialadenectomy ranges between 0% and 11% but hasdecreased in recent years to less than 5%.[16,18] Complications with transoral sialolithotomy, such as stenosis of the neo-ostium, damage to the lingual nerve, and ranula formation, are reported to occur at a rate of 4%. Sialadenectomy had an observed incidence of 1% to 3% with open transoral sialolithotomy.[20,21]

Significant costs are associated with sialendoscopes. A complete set of salivary endoscopes along with applicable dilators, hand drills, and microforceps cost up to $20,000 to $50,000, depending on the region.[14,15] Maintenance and repair costs could significantly compound this further, which, in the experience of this article's principal author, was approximately $60,000 during his first year of practice. In comparison, transoral sialolithotomy does not have a significant startup cost. Transoral sialolithotomy requires instruments available in an average oral tumor tray, which is readily available in most centers, whereas successful sialendoscopy often requires a variety of disposable instruments including guidewires, dilators, and baskets, which cost up to hundreds of dollars per use. A study in New Zealand found that the cost of transoral sialolithotomy per case was significantly less at NZ$409 (US$277) compared with NZ$638 (US$432) for sialendoscopy.[20]

Both sialendoscopy and transoral sialolithotomy have learning curves. Luers and colleagues[25] have shown that a surgeon in training required 30 cases to reach satisfactory operation times and performance ratings, reaching only a level of excellence in the last group of his 50 patients. Transoral sialolithotomy also presented with a potential learning curve; although, it is unclear how many surgeries are needed in order to attain adequate expertise in this procedure.[20]

An additional important point of comparison is the average case time for each modality. It is longer and highly variable for sialendoscopy at 71 ± 41 minutes, whereas transoral sialolithotomy reportedly takes an average of 28 minutes (25 ± 10.50 minutes for smaller sialoliths and 35 ± 16 minutes for larger ones).[20,26] These shorter case times for transoral sialolithotomy have the benefits of maximizing surgeon operative times, especially those in training, and optimize surgical resources, which ultimately reduces costs.

Finally, due to the combined cost and need of significant training, sialendoscopy is not readily available in certain regions. This limits patient accessibility compelling patients to seek care at tertiary centers, farther away from their residences. **Table 1** summarizes comparisons between sialendoscopy and transoral sialolithotomy.

TRANSORAL SIALOLITHOTOMY: A PROPOSED ALGORITHM

Obstructive salivary symptoms should first be evaluated with an imaging modality[14,20,23] (**Fig. 1**). Ultrasound may be performed if readily available, but CT should be used if the former cannot reliably rule out stones. Imaging characteristics should be used to evaluate whether to proceed to sialendoscopy or transoral sialolithotomy. Parotid gland stones should proceed with sialendoscopy or combined (open/endoscopic) techniques. Transoral sialolithotomy is indicated for submandibular sialolithiases that are either palpable or CT- or ultrasound-visualized, nonmobile, and greater than 5 mm. Sialoliths that are less than 5 mm should be evaluated for characteristics and location. Stones that are irregularly shaped have a higher risk for duct trauma or perforation with endoscopic removal; therefore, intraoperative conversion to transoral

Table 1 Comparison of sialendoscopy versus transoral sialolithotomy		
	Sialendoscopy	Transoral Sialolithotomy
Success rates	86%–93% (meta-analysis)	90%–95% (case series)
Average stone size	<5 mm	≥5 mm
Complication rates	2%–3%	3%–4%
Rate of sialadenectomy	0%–11%	1%–3%
Start-up cost	US$20,000-$50,000	US$1000–2000
Cost per case	US$432	US$277
Average case time	71 min	28 min
Availability	Mostly in tertiary centers	More accessible instrumentation; more widespread availability
Indications	Smaller (<5 mm) and mobile sialoliths; other causes of benign obstructive salivary disease (eg, strictures)	Palpable, ultrasound-/CT-visualized sialoliths larger than 5 mm
Contraindications	Active sialadenitis, complete distal duct stenosis, symptomatic intraparenchymal stone	Active sialadenitis, limited mouth opening

sialolithotomy may be indicated. Distal (anterior) Wharton duct stones are readily accessible by the surgeon; thus, such stones can often be removed via a transoral incision under local anesthesia in an office setting. Small (<5 mm), mobile, or oval-shaped sialoliths located between the submandibular hilum and the salivary ostia may be removed with sialendoscopic extraction, depending on surgeon preference and experience.

TRANSORAL SIALOLITHOTOMY: CONTRAINDICATIONS AND LIMITATIONS

Transoral sialolithotomy should not be performed in patients with acute sialadenitis.[20,27,28] Edema and inflammation in the area make visualization of the anatomy difficult, increasing the risk of complications such as ranula formation, lingual nerve injury, or spread of infection to the deep neck tissues. Limited mouth opening is also a contraindication, as safe access to the duct would be difficult to establish.

Currently, this should be limited to submandibular sialolithiasis in general otolaryngology practices. There is insufficient evidence for the effectiveness and safety of the procedure for sublingual sialoliths that carry a higher risk of postoperative ranula; thus, sublingual sialoliths may require sublingual gland excision. Although transoral sialolithotomy in parotid stones has been documented, significant morbidity has also been reported, such as transient facial nerve upper buccal branch palsies and the common complication of completion of stenosis of the parotid ostium. Therefore, transoral parotid duct sialolithotomy should be reserved for cases of failed sialendoscopic retrieval as a combined endoscopic-open technique due to the smaller diameter of Stensen duct.

TRANSORAL SIALOLITHOMY: A CASE PRESENTATION
History of Present Illness

A 54-year-old man presents with a history of intermittent swelling below the right jawline over the course of several years. These episodes would occur generally when eating, resolving within 20 to 30 minutes with neck massage. Six weeks ago,

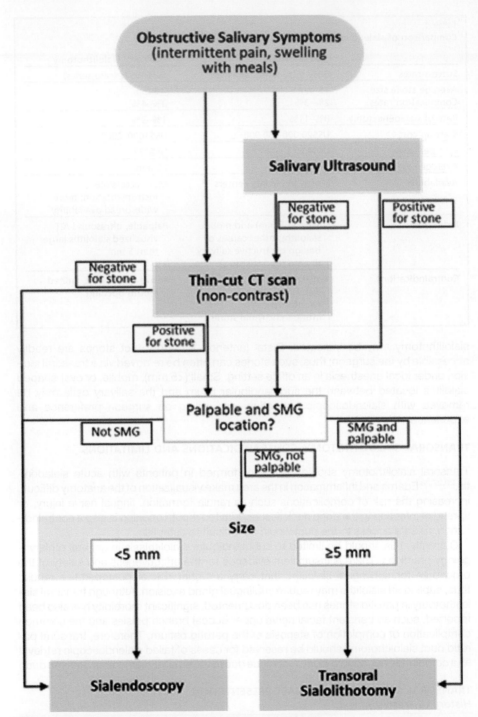

Fig. 1. A proposed algorithm for submandibular sialolithiasis.

he experienced acute swelling and tenderness in the area with foul-tasting saliva and mild redness of the neck. He was seen at a local clinic that started a course of oral antibiotics and corticosteroids, which resolved the pain and swelling within a few days. However, since that time he feels that the area is persistently swollen and worsens with additional swelling during meals. He has tried to manage this with increased hydration, sour candies, and warm compresses without relief. He denies swelling in any other neck location.

Past Medical History

The patient is healthy with no history of dry eyes, dry mouth, smoking, or the use of drying medications (eg, antihistamines, anticholinergics, diuretics, psychiatric medications). He drinks 2 cups of coffee in the morning. He gives no history of autoimmune disorders in the family or himself.

Physical Examination

The right submandibular gland is firm, enlarged, and nontender. There is no other adenopathy noted. Examination of the floor of mouth reveals thick mucoid saliva from the right Wharton papilla adjacent to the frenulum of the tongue. Bimanual palpation demonstrates a hard mass in the posterior floor of mouth. Right hemi-tongue sensation is intact on pinprick examination.

Differential Diagnosis

- Obstructive salivary disorder (stone, scar, foreign body)

Less likely:

- Nonobstructive salivary disorder (Sjögren, sarcoid)
- Recurrent salivary cyst/sialocele
- Salivary neoplasm

Imaging

Ultrasound of the right submandibular gland: an office-based ultrasonography demonstrates a right submandibular stone of 7 mm at the hilum of the gland superior to the mylohyoid muscle (**Fig. 2**). The stone is confirmed by bimanual palpation in which it is held between the tip of the examining gloved finger and the ultrasound probe. Because of confirmation of a stone on ultrasound, CT scan is not necessary but is an option for further confirmation (**Fig. 3**).

Management

The patient will benefit from surgical removal of the stone. Although acute infections can respond to antibiotic therapy, once a stone has caused an associated acute infection, it will remain a colonized biomass.

This colonized biomass has the potential for recurrent and progressive infections that can result in glandular abscess or deep neck infection. In addition, sialoliths typically grow over time (mean: 1 mm per year).

The patient can be presented with the following surgical options:

- *Right submandibular gland excision*: although this approach is an option, it has lost favor to less invasive techniques due to the potential for external scar, marginal mandibular nerve and lingual nerve weakness, loss of neck volume and change in contour, and loss of gland function. As a result, most experienced salivary centers reserve submandibular resection for cases of recurrent obstruction

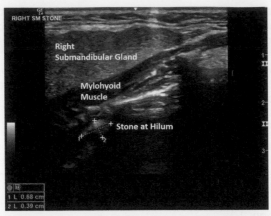

Fig. 2. Ultrasound showing a 7-mm stone at the hilum of the right submandibular gland.

after prior gland-preserving therapy or intraglandular or nonpalpable stones located inferior to the mylohyoid (approximately 5% of cases).

- *Gland-preserving approach*: using current techniques, salivary stones can be removed surgically 95% of the time while preserving the underlying gland. Small stones less than 5 mm in size can often be removed with endoscopy alone, whereas stones greater than 5 mm such as this one generally require a transoral sialolithotomy approach. There is the option to consent the patient for conversion to gland excision during the same procedure if the stone cannot be removed transorally or in the event of complete duct avulsion. Converting to gland excision after an unsuccessful transoral approach theoretically increases the risk of a salivary fistula although this is rarely observed in practice.The patient consents to transoral sialolithotomy.

Operative Technique

The procedure is performed in an outpatient ambulatory surgery center or hospital. Distal (anterior floor of mouth) stone extractions can be performed under local

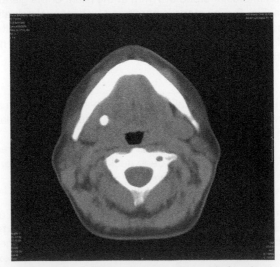

Fig. 3. CT image of 7-mm stone at hilum of right submandibular gland.

anesthesia with sedation. However, general anesthesia is preferable in most cases in order to maximize patient comfort, reduce patient motion, and reduce the chance of choking or aspirating blood and irrigation. The patient is nasally intubated in order to allow better visualization of the floor of mouth. Muscle relaxant is helpful to maximize mouth opening with a bite block or retractor. Intravenous dexamethasone reduces floor of mouth edema in the immediate postoperative period. A plastic cheek retractor, surgical loupes, and an adequate headlight improve visualization of the surgical field (**Fig. 4**). The hemi-tongue can be moved medially with a suture stitch or Sweetheart retractor. The surgeon should survey the surface anatomy of the floor of mouth in order to identify the bulge of the sublingual gland and/or uncinate process of the submandibular gland (the portion of the gland extending above the mylohyoid muscle) and the outline of the lingual nerve as it descends medial to the retromolar trigone into the floor of mouth. The target stone is palpated with bimanual examination in order to identify the location of the stone in the floor of mouth. A repeat ultrasound can be performed intraoperatively if the stone is not palpable or has changed location since the prior examination.

Once the surgeon has a mental image of the stone location, a linear 2- to 3-cm incision is made through the floor of mouth mucosa overlying the stone location medial to the hump of glandular mass using a needle tip electrocautery in cut mode. Care is taken not to extend the incision into deeper tissues. Gentle blunt dissection with a tonsil clamp or mosquito allows identification of underlying structures such as gland, lingual nerve, and Wharton duct. The duct is typically a grayish tubular structure that extends along the medial border of the gland (sublingual or uncinated process of the

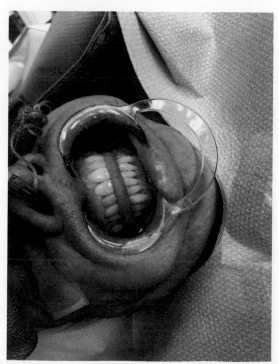

Fig. 4. Nasal intubation and plastic cheek retractor to provide excellent exposure to the floor of mouth.

submandibular gland). Vicryl (4.0) sutures can be placed through the mucosal and submucosal tissues and used to retract the incision. Once the duct is identified, a vessel loop is placed around the duct for gentle forward retraction (**Fig. 5**). The duct is followed posteriorly toward the gland with gentle dissection of the overlying tissues and extension of the incision if needed. The lingual nerve should be identified as it descends lateral to the duct and crosses deep to the duct in a lateral to medial direction. Occasionally the lingual nerve will need to be encircled with a second vessel loop to allow lateral retraction in order to visualize the hilum of the gland. At this point, a surgical assistant should push the submandibular gland up toward the floor of mouth externally as the surgeon performs additional intraoral palpation to confirm the stone location. Although the assistant is pushing upward, and the surgeon is gently pulling the duct anteriorly with the vessel loop, the stone will appear as a yellow or whitish mass within the duct. A linear incision can be through the duct directly onto the stone using the needle tip electrocautery, or alternatively the duct can be opened on its superior surface from distal to proximal using ball-tipped scissors (Video 1). Once the stone is visualized, a Rosen needle or fine pick can be used to tease it out of the duct and pass it off the field. The dichotomy can then be rinsed with saline irrigation using a 20-gauge angiocatheter, which will dislodge inflammatory debris or small stone fragments. If feasible, several 4.0-vicryl sutures can be used to tack the duct wall to the posterior floor of mouth. If this is not allowed, the overlying mucosa can be closed loosely with interrupted 4.0-vicryl suture, which has not been observed to increase the risk of postoperative obstruction. Ductal stents are not required. The cheek and jaw retractors are removed. The occlusion is checked to ensure that the temporomandibular joint was not dislocated during the case.

Postoperative Care

The patient may resume a soft or normal diet immediately. The patient is asked to rinse with warm saline or chlorhexidine gluconate oral rinse after meals. The patient should take care to drink plenty of fluids and massage the gland in the weeks after the

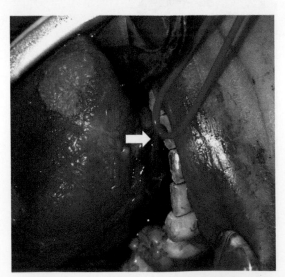

Fig. 5. Vessel loop provides gentle traction on Wharton duct, which pulls the area of blockage forward to within view (*Arrow* indicates Wharton's duct).

procedure in order to maintain salivary flow through the neo-ostium. A 1-week course of oral antibiotics (amoxicillin/clavulanate or clindamycin) and oral steroid taper pack reduces local tissue inflammation and promote wound healing.

A postoperative appointment is made for 3 to 4 weeks after surgery to allow for a wound check and assessment of symptom resolution. If the patient is doing well with resolution of symptoms within 1 month of surgery, they are unlikely to require ongoing follow-up. Up to one-third of patients will have some ongoing salivary obstruction after surgery, most likely due to ductal scar; however, these symptoms are generally mild and much improved compared with preoperative symptoms.[29] If significant obstruction returns, the patient will require evaluation for retained or recurrent stone or obstructive scar tissue that may require surgical revision.

Complications

Swelling of the floor of the mouth and affected submandibular gland with disturbance in swallowing may occasionally occur in the postoperative period; however, it is rare to have to admit a patient for inpatient observation following the procedure.

Potential complications with transoral sialolithotomy are fortunately rare. A missed or retained stone can occur in 5% of cases. A retained stone may lead to gland or deep neck abscess if ongoing symptoms are present. Therefore, revision surgery for symptomatic stones is advised. If the patient remains symptom free, an asymptomatic stone or fragment can be observed over time with intervention held until the onset of symptoms.

Temporary paresthesias of the lingual nerve are common but generally resolve within a few weeks of surgery. Permanent damage to the lingual nerve is rare occurring in less than 1% of cases. Other complications include stenosis of the neo-ostium, ranula formation, and postoperative infection. These types of complications occur at a rate of about 3% to 4%. The need for submandibulectomy due to inability to remove the stone and/or complete ductal avulsion is required in less than 2% of cases.

SUMMARY

Although sialendoscopy has obvious utility in many obstructive salivary diseases, including small and multiple stones, strictures, and inflammatory/autoimmune disorders, transoral sialolithotomy without endoscopy is safe, effective, and economic for sialolithiasis with a definable target (fixed and palpable). This approach provides a more accessible intervention for patients, especially those who are far from tertiary care centers with sialendoscopy instrumentation and experienced surgeons.

CLINICS CARE POINTS

- Imaging studies are indicated for obstructive salivary symptoms such as intermittent pain and swelling with meals by ultrasound if readily available and/or CT scan.
- If these imaging modalities are negative for stones, patients should be referred for sialendoscopy to evaluate for strictures, fibrosis, or radiotransparent/small stones.
- When any imaging modality yields positive for stone, sialoliths should be characterized by their palpability, location, and size to determine whether to proceed with sialendoscopy or transoral sialolithotomy.
- Transoral sialolithotomy may be performed with intraoperative ultrasound to guide the surgeon but is not necessary when the stone is readily palpable.

DISCLOSURE

The authors have nothing to disclose.

SUPPLEMENTARY DATA

Supplementary data related to this article can be found online at https://doi.org/10. 1016/j.otc.2021.01.006.

REFERENCES

1. Sigismund PE, Zenk J, Koch M, et al. Nearly 3,000 salivary stones: Some clinical and epidemiologic aspects. Laryngoscope 2015;125(8):1879–82.
2. Escudier MP, McGurk M. Symptomatic sialoadenitis and sialolithiasis in the English population, an estimate of the cost of hospital treatment. Br Dent J 1999; 186(9):463–6.
3. Rzymska-Grala I, Stopa Z, Grala B, et al. Salivary gland calculi - contemporary methods of imaging. Pol J Radiol 2010;75(3):25–37.
4. Harrison JD. Causes, natural history, and incidence of salivary stones and obstructions. Otolaryngol Clin North Am 2009;42(6):927–47. Table of Contents.
5. Marchal F, Kurt AM, Dulguerov P, et al. Retrograde theory in sialolithiasis formation. Arch Otolaryngol Head Neck Surg 2001;127(1):66–8.
6. Marchal F, Dulguerov P. Sialolithiasis management: The state of the art. Arch Otolaryngol Head Neck Surg 2003;129(9):951–6.
7. Ilgit ET, Çizmeli MO, Işik S, et al. Digital subtraction sialography: technique, advantages and results in 107 cases. Eur J Radiol 1992;15(3):244–7.
8. Hammett JT, Walker C. Sialolithiasis. In: StatPearls. Treasure Island (FL): StatPearls Publishing; 2020. Available at: https://www.statpearls.com/.
9. Terraz S, Poletti PA, Dulguerov P, et al. How reliable is sonography in the assessment of sialolithiasis? AJR Am J Roentgenol 2013;201(1):W104–9.
10. Thomas WW, Douglas JE, Rassekh CH. Accuracy of Ultrasonography and Computed Tomography in the Evaluation of Patients Undergoing Sialendoscopy for Sialolithiasis. Otolaryngol Head Neck Surg 2017;156(5):834–9.
11. Katz P. [Endoscopy of the salivary glands]. Ann Radiol 1991;34(1–2):110–3.
12. Marchal F, Kurt AM, Dulguerov P, et al. Histopathology of submandibular glands removed for sialolithiasis. Ann Otol Rhinol Laryngol 2001;110(5 Pt 1):464–9.
13. Su YX, Xu JH, Liao GQ, et al. Salivary gland functional recovery after sialendoscopy. Laryngoscope 2009;119(4):646–52.
14. Fabie JE, Kompelli AR, Naylor TM, et al. Gland-preserving surgery for salivary stones and the utility of sialendoscopes. Head Neck 2019;41(5):1320–7.
15. Felton M, Mamais C, Kumar BN, et al. Medico-legal aspects of introducing sialendoscopy: A minimally invasive treatment for salivary gland obstruction. Clin Otolaryngol 2012;37(3):213–20.
16. Nahlieli O. Complications of sialendoscopy: personal experience, literature analysis, and suggestions. J Oral Maxillfac Surg 2015;73(1):75–80.
17. Al-Abri R, Marchal F. New era of endoscopic approach for sialolithiasis: sialendoscopy. Sultan Qaboos Univ Med J 2010;10(3):382–7.
18. Strychowsky JE, Sommer DD, Gupta MK, et al. Sialendoscopy for the management of obstructive salivary gland disease: a systematic review and meta-analysis. Arch Otolaryngol Head Neck Surg 2012;138(6):541–7.
19. Iro H, Zenk J, Escudier MP, et al. Outcome of minimally invasive management of salivary calculi in 4,691 patients. Laryngoscope 2009;119(2):263–8.

20. Shashinder S, Morton R, Ahmad Z. Outcome and relative cost of transoral removal of submandibular calculi. J Laryngol Otol 2011;125:386-9.
21. Zenk J, Constantinidis J, Al-Kadah B, et al. Transoral removal of submandibular stones. Arch Otolaryngol Head Neck Surg 2001;127(4):432-6.
22. Park JS, Sohn JH, Kim JK. Factors influencing intraoral removal of submandibular calculi. Otolaryngol Head Neck Surg 2006;135(5):704-9.
23. Juul ML, Wagner N. Objective and subjective outcome in 42 patients after treatment of sialolithiasis by transoral incision of Warthon's duct: a retrospective middle-term follow-up study. Eur Arch Otorhinolaryngol 2014;271(11):3059-66.
24. Zenk J, Koch M, Klintworth N, et al. Sialendoscopy in the diagnosis and treatment of sialolithiasis: a study on more than 1000 patients. Otolaryngol Head Neck Surg 2012;147(5):858-63.
25. Luers JC, Damm M, Klussmann JP, et al. The learning curve of sialendoscopy with modular sialendoscopes: a single surgeon's experience. Arch Otolaryngol Head Neck Surg 2010;136(8):762-5.
26. Marchal F, Barki G, Dulguerov P, et al. Submandibular diagnostic and interventional sialendoscopy: new procedure for ductal disorders. Ann Otol Rhinol Laryngol 2002;111(1):27-35.
27. Foletti J-M, Wajszczak L, Gormezano M, et al. Transoral Stensen's Duct Approach: A 22-case retrospective study. J Craniomaxillofac Surg 2016;44(11):1796-9.
28. Gallo A, Benazzo M, Capaccio P, et al. Sialoendoscopy: state of the art, challenges and further perspectives. Round Table, 101(st) SIO National Congress, Catania 2014. Acta Otorhinolaryngol Ital 2015;35(4):217-33.
29. Gillespie MB, O'Connell BP, Rawl JW, et al. Clinical and quality-of-life outcomes following gland-preserving surgery for chronic sialadenitis. Laryngoscope 2015;125:1340-4.

Soft Tissue Reconstruction of Parotidectomy Defect

Jennifer Moy, MD, Mark K. Wax, MD, FRCS(C), Myriam Loyo, MD, MCR*

KEYWORDS

- Parotidectomy • Reconstruction • Fat graft • Alloderm • Frey syndrome • Free flap

KEY POINTS

- Parotidectomy creates a soft tissue defect for which reconstruction will improve both facial contour and patient satisfaction.
- Postoperative Frey syndrome (gustatory sweating) can be prevented with soft tissue reconstruction by creating a barrier to aberrant reinnervation of the cheek skin.
- Acellular dermis, autologous fat transfer with/without dermis, and local/regional flaps are used for reconstruction for most defects of the parotid bed.
- For extensive composite large volume or surface area defects, consider free tissue transfer.

INTRODUCTION

Surgical resection of parotid tumors leads to a loss in lateral facial volume, resulting in a noticeable facial deformity with asymmetry. This defect can vary from a small posterior mandibular depression to significant facial concavity. In larger composite defects, the loss of volume may cause inferior displacement and medial rotation of the auricle. In a study of patients having undergone parotidectomy, 70% reported a change in appearance, with greater than half reporting a noticeable depression. Furthermore, casual observers notice this contour defect.[1,2] Facial appearance and deformity is a critical aspect affecting quality of life and carries strong social penalties.[3] Multiple studies have shown facial deformities affect attractiveness, self-esteem, academic and occupational satisfaction, income, and quality of life. Because patients may be concerned regarding facial contour after parotidectomy, soft tissue reconstruction can normalize facial appearance and decrease the psychosocial impacts with an overall increase in patient satisfaction.[4,5]

In addition to restoring facial contour, postoperative Frey syndrome can be prevented with soft tissue reconstruction. Frey syndrome, or gustatory sweating, is the postparotidectomy phenomenon where sweating occurs in the skin of the cheek while eating. It is attributed to aberrant reinnervation of parotid parasympathetic nerve fibers

Department of Otolaryngology/Head and Neck Surgery at Oregon Health & Science University, 3181 SW Sam Jackson Park Road, PV01, Portland, OR 97239, USA
* Corresponding author.
E-mail address: loyo@ohsu.edu

Otolaryngol Clin N Am 54 (2021) 567–581
https://doi.org/10.1016/j.otc.2021.02.009
0030-6665/21/© 2021 Elsevier Inc. All rights reserved.

oto.theclinics.com

to the sympathetic fibers in the skin of the cheek. The manifestations can develop years after parotidectomy. Although this phenomenon is reported by 38% of patients, objective testing for Frey syndrome using the minor starch-iodine test shows that up to 96% of patients have this phenomenon after parotidectomy without reconstruction.[6] Surgical reconstruction can prevent Frey syndrome by creating a barrier between the parasympathetic nerves of the parotid bed and the overlying skin. This barrier can be created with local flaps, fat grafts, acellular dermal matrix, or free tissue transfer.

This chapter discusses soft tissue reconstruction options for the parotidectomy defect, including wound healing, Frey syndrome, and tumor surveillance.

SKIN INCISION

The modified Blair incision (**Fig. 1**A) is widely used as an approach for parotid surgery. A reliable incision camouflages well and provides good exposure of the mastoid tip,

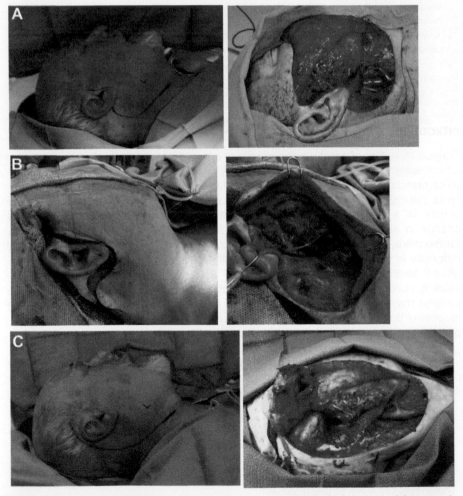

Fig. 1. Skin incisions. (*A*) Modified Blair incision; (*B*) modified facelift incision; (*C*) postauricular incision.

sternocleidomastoid and posterior digastric belly muscles, and the entire parotid gland. Alternatively, the modified facelift incision (**Fig. 1**B) obviates the neck incision yet provides similar exposure. The modified facelift incision is associated with improved patient satisfaction without an increase in surgical time or complications.[7,8] Caution should be taken in large, anterior tumors, where retrograde dissection of the facial nerve may be required, as this approach may not provide safe exposure.[7] The contraindications described in the literature are tumors with parapharyngeal space extension, recurrent tumors, and arteriovenous malformation.[9]

When a lateral or subtotal temporal bone resection with or without auriculectomy is performed, a postauricular incision [**Fig. 1**C] is made and carried anteroinferiorly to a neck skin crease.

Reconstructive Options

The volume of removed parotid tissue, the individual patient's facial anatomy, and the patient's desires and values should be considered in choosing a reconstruction technique. Reconstructive options range from primary closure, fat or acellular implants to locoregional flaps, and free tissue transfer. **Table 1** summarizes each reconstructive option, with indications, advantages, disadvantages, and surgical tips.

Primary closure is an excellent option for most superficial parotidectomy defects with minimal-to-no skin loss. Wide undermining of the soft tissue deep to the superficial musculoaponeurotic system (SMAS) allows plication and prevents excessive tension on the skin edges. The scalp does not offer the same laxity as the face and neck for assisting in primary closure. However, galeal-releasing incisions made at 1-cm intervals can provide some additional reach while maintaining adequate blood supply to the skin edge. A tension-free repair is especially important in an irradiated field where there is a propensity for wound healing complications.

Acellular dermal implants, such as AlloDerm (LifeCell Corporation, Branchburg, New Jersey) and DermaMatrix (Synthes Corporation, Westchester, Pennsylvania), are off-the-shelf and ready-to-use sheets derived from human cadaveric skin (**Fig. 2**). Because of their availability, simplicity, and lack of donor site morbidity, acellular dermal implants are a favored reconstructive option for limited parotidectomy defects, despite concerns for these materials increasing the risk of seroma and sialocele.[10] A meta-analysis of 5 clinical controlled studies showed acellular dermal implants significantly reduced the rate of Frey syndrome and salivary leaks without an increase in wound complications.[11] Use of a single sheet allows for the best healing potential, whereas using more than one sheet can increase local wound complications, limiting the degree of contour improvement that can be achieved. Although contour improvement is underreported, a randomized controlled trial of 36 patients undergoing parotidectomy compared acellular dermis with free fat grafting. This study showed free fat reconstruction resulted in better aesthetic outcomes, and lower cost and complication rates,[12] suggesting a limitation in the degree of augmentation attainable with AlloDerm. AlloDerm has been more widely used for parotidectomy reconstruction than DermaMatrix. Limited studies directly comparing these materials are available.[10]

Fat grafting is a popular reconstructive option for parotidectomy defects, given its simplicity, limited donor morbidity, and generally satisfactory outcomes. Fat grafting improves facial symmetry and reduces the incidence of Frey syndrome with better patient satisfaction scores.[4,13–15] This technique has been used in tumors ranging in size from less than 1 to 7 cm and with volumes of up to 70 cm.[3,4,14,16,17] Fat grafts are harvested either as a free graft or as a dermal graft from the abdomen or thigh. Free fat grafts are typically harvested from the periumbilical fat, through a well-hidden incision in the lower half of the umbilicus.[4] Harvesting a single generous piece of abdominal fat

Table 1
Pros and cons of reconstructive option

	Indicated Defect	Advantages	Disadvantages	Surgical Tips
Primary closure	Superficial parotidectomies, tail of parotid	No donor morbidity, short OR time	Only for small defects, wound healing concerns for postradiated wounds	Wide undermining, SMAS plicating, and galeal releasing incisions can help create a tension-free skin closure
Acellular dermal implant	Superficial parotidectomies, tail of parotid	No donor morbidity, short OR time	Cost	Limit to 1 sheet of implant to prevent complications
Fat graft	Superficial parotidectomies, tail of parotid, deep lobe	Low-donor site morbidity, similar consistency to parotid tissue, limited additional operative time	Risk of fat necrosis, infection, and fat reabsorption	Harvest as a single-large piece; overcorrect 10%–30% in anticipation of atrophy, consider a dermal fat graft to reduce atrophy
Local and regional grafts	Deep/total parotidectomy, skin defects	Excellent skin match	Reach can be limited, wound healing concerns in postirradiated fields	Inferiorly based flaps require strategically placed tacking sutures to prevent flap ptosis and dehiscence
Cervicofacial rotational flap	Skin defects	Excellent skin match with low donor site morbidity	Lacks tridimensional volume restoration	Can extend onto chest to gain additional reach
Temporalis muscle/temporoparietal fascia flap	Superior defects without skin involvement	Short OR time	Donor site defect, limited reach inferiorly, relies on intact superficial temporal vessels, risk to frontal branch of the facial nerve	
Sternomastoid myofacial flap	Tail of parotid, mastoid defects	Minimal morbidity, similar intraoperative exposure, short OR time	Limited reach, added risk to CN XI	Use caution with concurrent neck dissection to prevent loss of blood supply

Pectoralis myofacial or myocutaneous flap	Deep/total parotidectomy, skin defects	Reliable flap with good bulk	Donor site morbidity	Place superiorly placed tacking sutures to prevent ptosis, can add length by dissecting muscle away from pedicle as muscle heads to humerus. Most common with auriculectomies
Latissimus dorsi myofacial or myocutaneous flap	Deep/total parotidectomy, skin defects	Large, thin muscle that can be contoured in defect, low donor site morbidity	Poor skin match, added OR time	Place superiorly placed tacking sutures to prevent ptosis. Most commonly used with auriculectomies
Keystone island flap	Deep/total parotidectomy, skin defects	Excellent skin match with low donor site morbidity	Lacks tridimensional volume restoration	Can be harvested posterosuperiorly based on occipital and posterior auricular perforators, anterioinferiorly based on the facial or submental perforators, or inferiorly based on the transverse cervical or superficial cervical arteries
Submental island flap	Deep/total parotidectomy, skin defects	Excellent skin match with low donor site morbidity	Requires intact facial vessels, limited bulk	Harvest with underlying muscles for added strength and bulk
Supraclavicular island flap	Deep/total parotidectomy, skin defects	Excellent skin match with low donor site morbidity	Can be folded on itself to provide adequate bulk	Most common complication is wound dehiscence, therefore placating deep dermal sutures to ensure a tension-free skin closure is imperative

(continued on next page)

Table 1
(continued)

	Indicated Defect	Advantages	Disadvantages	Surgical Tips
Free tissue transfer	Total parotidectomy, skin defects, chemo/radiation	Highly vascularized to withstand chemotherapy and radiation	Increased OR time, donor site morbidity	Can be deepithelialized and buried for bulk
Radial forearm	Skin defect, with minimal volume loss	Long pedicle length, reliable, no atrophy	Lacks bulk, donor site morbidity, requires skin graft	Can be deepithelialized and buried for bulk or by including upper forearm subcutaneous fat
Anterolateral thigh	Total parotidectomy, skin defects, chemo/radiation	Excellent bulk that can be modified to accommodate defect and cover vital structures, relatively low morbidity	Short pedicle length, can be too bulky in overweight/obese patients	Ability to include fascia lata for static facial reanimation and/or vastus lateralis with its motor nerve to be grafted for dynamic facial reanimation

Abbreviations: CN, cranial nerve; OR, operating room.

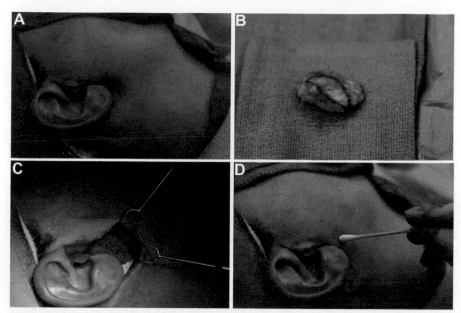

Fig. 2. Dermal fat grafting. (*A*) Retromandibular concavity following parotidectomy; (*B*) dermal fat graft, with deepithelialized dermis outlined in black ink; (*C*) inset of fat graft; (*D*) improvement of contour defect following dermal fat graft.

is preferred over multiple small grafts, as it minimizes graft trauma and devascularization, which may lead to increased graft necrosis and loss. Dermal fat grafts (**Fig. 3**) theoretically support vascularization of the fat through the subdermal plexus. Dermal fat grafts are harvested from the lower abdomen with a Pfannenstiel incision below the bikini line.[13,18,19] One advantage of a dermal fat graft is that the subdermal tissue can

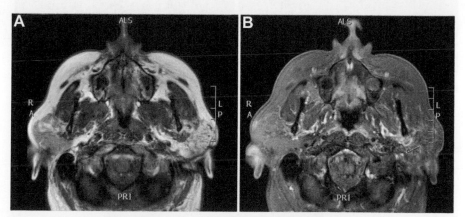

Fig. 3. MRI postparotidectomy with dermal fat graft. Right parotid gland has normal appearance. The left side is post–total parotidectomy with mastoidectomy and dermal fat grafting for recurrent pleomorphic adenoma. (*A*) Axial T1-weighted without contrast; (*B*) axial T1-weighted with fat suppression. Residual disease is easily delineated from surrounding fat graft (*arrow*).

readily be sutured to allow for better positioning of the graft in the defect. High patient and surgeon satisfaction with the reconstructive contour and the donor site have been reported for both techniques of fat grafting[16,17,19,20]; however, studies directly comparing free fat grafts with dermal fat grafts are not available.

Local wound complications after fat graft reconstruction of the parotidectomy are rare. Hematomas, seromas, and wound infections can occur at both the donor and the reconstructive sites.[4,16,17] Fat necrosis can lead to infection, which may improve with antibiotics and local wound care. In more severe cases, fat necrosis may require graft removal. Although rare, epithelial cysts can develop in dermal fat grafts if the epidermis is not carefully removed.[19] The primary downside of fat grafting is variable reabsorption over time. Most surgeons recommend overcorrecting volume loss by 10% to 30%.[4,12,17,18,21] Although the fat graft stabilizes after 6 months, it can be debulked if overcorrection persists.[16] Some investigators speculate using a SMAS flap can improve the viability of the fat graft and decrease resorption[17]; however, studies that objectively measure graft survival over time are lacking. A limited case series reviewed 5 cases of postparotidectomy/fat graft MRI showing stable graft volume 1 to 3 years after implantation.[22]

Historically, there has been concern that reconstructive techniques can obstruct the ability to assess tumor recurrence.[14] However, advanced imaging techniques, computed tomography, MRI, and PET imaging can reliably delineate between normal reconstructive and parotid tissues from tumor recurrence (**Fig. 4**).[4,22] Although some investigators advocate waiting 6 months to 2 years,[19] several have published successful use of fat grafting in parotid malignancy reconstruction.[4,14,17]

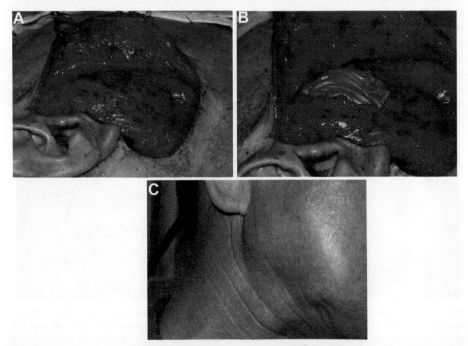

Fig. 4. Alloderm reconstruction. (*A*) Anterior parotid defect; (*B*) alloderm implant into defect, (*C*) postoperative outcome with lack of facial concavity.

Local and Regional Flaps

Local and regional flaps, including myofascial, myocutaneous, and fasciocutaneous flaps, are particularly useful in small to moderate defects. In cases in which skin restoration is necessary, they provide excellent skin color match with lower distant morbidity. They are well vascularized, allowing longer random pattern paddles with smaller pedicles than would be allowed elsewhere in the body. However, they do require incision planning with the ablative surgeons and often lack adequate bulk to provide good facial contour in larger resections. Because of decreased vascularization and fibrosis, rotational flaps are not ideal for moderate to large defects in postirradiated patients.

The SMAS can be used as a local muscle flap to assist in volume replacement and reduction of Frey syndrome incidence. When the SMAS is mobilized, advanced, and plicated posteriorly into the defect, it can be used for volume restoration. However, facial asymmetry may result from significant unilateral plication, necessitating contralateral SMAS rhytidectomy.[23] Because of its thin nature and limited volume, the SMAS may not be available in all cases, especially in superficial tumors where resection of this layer is required for adequate margins.

The *cervicofacial rotation flap* can cover large skin defects with excellent skin color match (**Fig. 5**). Although it lacks tridimensionality, a concurrent muscle flap, such as temporalis, *sternocleidomastoid (SCM)*, or pectoralis can provide this bulk. The reliability of this flap is compromised by prior radiation, smoking, and sacrifice of the facial artery during resection or neck dissection. Because of its caudally based vascular supply, there is reduced survival and increased dehiscence above the zygoma. However, extension of the incision onto the chest improves reach and vascularity.

By extending the incision into the temporal region, the *temporalis muscle* and/or *temporoparietal fascia (TPF) flap* can be used as a rotational flap to provide soft tissue bulk to the parotid defect. Many argue against the use of the temporalis muscle flap for contour, as it results in temporal "hollowing," thus creating one defect to fix another. In addition, the temporalis muscle flap has limited reach beyond the mastoid.[24] Conversely, the TPF flap is thin, with excellent pliability that can provide coverage of the entire parotid bed, including the retromandibular area.[25] Although it has excellent vascularity, damage to the superficial temporal vessels during parotidectomy can

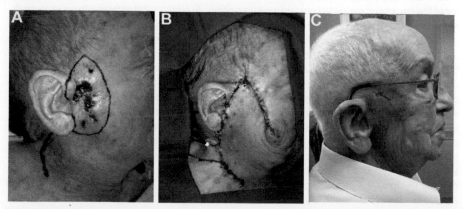

Fig. 5. Cervicofacial rotation flap. (*A*) Cutaneous carcinoma with planned incision drawn; (*B*) postablation with cervicofacial rotation flap; (*C*) six-month follow-up.

compromise the flap viability. Although these flaps have been shown to reduce the incidence of Frey syndrome to 8% from 43%, they have added risk to the frontal branch of the facial nerve, alopecia, hematoma, and increased operative time with less than optimal cosmetic reconstruction.[25]

The *SCM, pectoralis*, and *latissimus muscle flaps* can also be used as local rotational flaps to provide soft tissue restoration for the parotid defect. The SCM flap is harvested through the parotidectomy incision with improved bulk compared with the SMAS flap.[26] Several studies have failed to show improved facial contour after SCM flap,[26,27] whereas other studies have shown some degree of improvement.[28,29] The SCM flap can be harvested superiorly or inferiorly. A superiorly based flap is harvested from the superior third of the SCM, freed from the inferior attachment and rotated 180° around its anterior margin and sutured to the remnant parotid fascia or periosteum of the zygoma. The inferiorly based SCM flap is incised superiorly and anteriorly, then rotated into inferior and midparotid defects. The SCM flap has the potential to create a depression in the donor site and expose the spinal accessory nerve to damage.[28] An additional consideration in patients undergoing concurrent neck dissection is disrupting the tenuous blood supply to the SCM.

The pectoralis and latissimus flaps can be harvested as myocutaneous flaps to provide both bulk and cutaneous reconstruction if needed. These muscle flaps are usually reserved for parotidectomy defects with auriculectomy. The pectoralis flap carries significant donor site morbidity with poor contouring capability. The latissimus can be contoured more easily with the laxity of the posterior back skin allowing nearly all wounds to be closed primarily with minimal morbidity. When using inferiorly based rotational flaps, superior tacking sutures are important to prevent descent and dehiscence.

There has been great success in the use of various island flaps for the reconstruction of the parotidectomy defect. These include the *keystone, submental*, and *supraclavicular island flaps* (**Fig. 6**). Although they have excellent skin color match and low donor site morbidity, they lack 3-dimensional bulk for large contour defects.[30–32] Care must be taken in patients who have received preoperative radiation, concurrent neck dissection, or anticipate postoperative radiation.[32]

Free Tissue Transfer

In patients with large volume composite defects, recurrent tumor, dural defects, and prior irradiated fields or when postoperative radiation is anticipated, free tissue transfer is the most appropriate reconstructive option. Free flaps offer flexibility in size, bulk, reliability, and resilience. There are many donor site options for free flaps. The choice depends on the cutaneous tissue loss, contour defect, or exposed vital structures. The use of a deepithelialized buried free flap has been used with great success, with good facial contour, and vascularized soft tissue coverage of vital structures.[33]

The *radial forearm free flap (RFFF)* is a reliable flap with a long vascular pedicle that offers significant surface area coverage. It is limited by its modest bulk, depending on the habitus of the patient; thus, it is best suited for smaller defects with auricular preservation. However, additional bulk can be achieved if the upper forearm subcutaneous tissue is concurrently harvested. With deepithelialization, the flap can be placed within the parotid bed as a buried flap for contouring if there is no significant skin defect. The thin quality of the flap and lack of considerable change over time (ie muscle atrophy) obviates flap revision. However, closure of the donor site requires an additional skin graft, contributing to the morbidity in this flap. High-volume composite defects are best reconstructed with flaps containing muscle or a thick, soft tissue component.

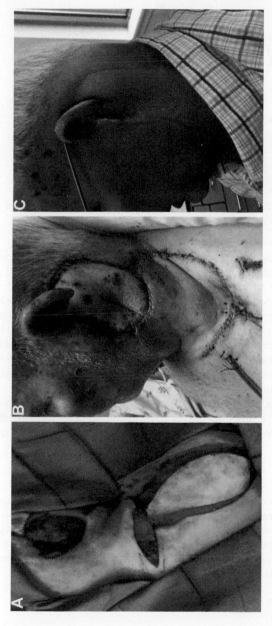

Fig. 6. Supraclavicular island flap. (*A*) Defect with supraclavicular island flap incised; (*B*) immediate postoperative reconstruction; (*C*) six-month follow-up.

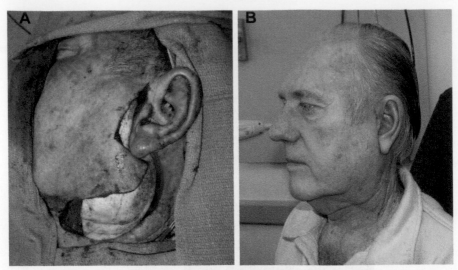

Fig. 7. Deepithelialized buried anterolateral thigh free flap. (*A*) Flap placed within parotid defect before deepithelialization; (*B*) six-month follow-up.

The *anterolateral thigh (ALT) free flap* is the ideal reconstructive option for large volume composite defects, especially with significant cutaneous loss and or lateral skull base resections with or without dural defects. The pedicle is based off the lateral circumflex femoral artery and can be up to 12 cm long. The skin paddle is limited to 8 to 12 cm in width to accommodate primary closure of the thigh, whereas the bulk of this flap largely depends on the gender and habitus of the patient. However, there are many options to choose from in the ALT flap in order to obtain ideal bulk, contour, and skin reconstruction. It can be harvested as a myofascial flap, to provide bulk, or a myocutaneous or fasciocutaneous flap to provide bulk and skin coverage. The ALT flap can be further deepithealialized for placement as a buried flap, if little to no skin defect is created (**Fig. 7**). Although this flap carries excellent resilience through postoperative radiation,[33] it has drawbacks such as the need for frequent debulking procedures, increased donor site seromas, and wound dehiscence when compared with the RFFF.[34,35]

SUMMARY

Soft tissue reconstruction of the parotidectomy defect can vary from primary closure to acellular dermal implants or fat grafts to local, regional, or free flaps. Many studies have shown improved facial contour, reduced incidence of Frey syndrome, and improved patient satisfaction with soft tissue reconstruction. Each reconstructive option carries specific indications, advantages, and risk. Patient anatomy and desires should be considered when selecting a reconstruction option.

CLINICS CARE POINTS

- Most parotidectomy defects can be successfully reconstructed with acellular matrix, fat grafts, or locoregional flaps with excellent patient satisfaction, reduced Frey syndrome, and minimal donor site morbidity.

- Fat grafts have a propensity to resorb, especially after radiation. Overcorrection, avoiding piece-meal harvesting, and/or using dermal fat or a local flap concurrently may reduce this phenomenon.

- Ensure to place superiorly placed tacking sutures on inferiorly based rotational flaps to prevent descent and dehiscence.

- Free tissue transfer is a superior option in large composite resections and when adjuvant radiation is expected.

DISCLOSURE

The authors have no disclosures.

REFERENCES

1. Nitzan D, Kronenberg J, Horowitz Z, et al. Quality of life following parotidectomy for malignant and benign disease. Plast Reconstr Surg 2004;114(5):1060–7.
2. Ciuman RR, Oels W, Jaussi R, et al. Outcome, general, and symptom-specific quality of life after various types of parotid resection. Laryngoscope 2012;122(6):1254–61.
3. Dey JK, Ishii M, Boahene KD, et al. Impact of facial defect reconstruction on attractiveness and negative facial perception. Laryngoscope 2015;125(6): 1316–21.
4. Conger BT, Gourin CG. Free abdominal fat transfer for reconstruction of the total parotidectomy defect. Laryngoscope 2008;118(7):1186–90.
5. Dey JK, Ishii LE, Byrne PJ, et al. The social penalty of facial lesions: new evidence supporting high-quality reconstruction. JAMA Facial Plast Surg 2015; 17(2):90–6.
6. Linder TE, Huber A, Schmid S. Frey's syndrome after parotidectomy: a retrospective and prospective analysis. Laryngoscope 1997;107(11 Pt 1):1496–501.
7. Grover N, D'Souza A. Facelift approach for parotidectomy: an evolving aesthetic technique. Otolaryngol Head Neck Surg 2013;148(4):548–56.
8. Bianchi B, Ferri A, Ferrari S, et al. Improving esthetic results in benign parotid surgery: statistical evaluation of facelift approach, sternocleidomastoid flap, and superficial musculoaponeurotic system flap application. J Oral Maxillofac Surg 2011;69(4):1235–41.
9. Terris DJ, Tuffo KM, Fee WE Jr. Modified facelift incision for parotidectomy. J Laryngol Otol 1994;108(7):574–8.
10. Athavale SM, Phillips S, Mangus B, et al. Complications of alloderm and dermamatrix for parotidectomy reconstruction. Head Neck 2012;34(1):88–93.
11. Zeng XT, Tang XJ, Wang XJ, et al. AlloDerm implants for prevention of Frey syndrome after parotidectomy: a systematic review and meta-analysis. Mol Med Rep 2012;5(4):974–80.
12. Wang S, Li L, Chen J, et al. Effects of free fat grafting on the prevention of Frey's syndrome and facial depression after parotidectomy: a prospective randomized trial. Laryngoscope 2016;126(4):815–9.
13. Harada T, Inoue T, Harashina T, et al. Dermis-fat graft after parotidectomy to prevent Frey's syndrome and the concave deformity. Ann Plast Surg 1993;31(5): 450–2.
14. Curry JM, Fisher KW, Heffelfinger RN, et al. Superficial musculoaponeurotic system elevation and fat graft reconstruction after superficial parotidectomy. Laryngoscope 2008;118(2):210–5.

15. Curry JM, King N, Reiter D, et al. Meta-analysis of surgical techniques for preventing parotidectomy sequelae. Arch Facial Plast Surg 2009;11(5): 327–31.

16. Loyo M, Gourin CG. Free abdominal fat transfer for partial and total parotidectomy defect reconstruction. Laryngoscope 2016;126(12):2694–8.

17. Ambro BT, Goodstein LA, Morales RE, et al. Evaluation of superficial musculoaponeurotic system flap and fat graft outcomes for benign and malignant parotid disease. Otolaryngol Head Neck Surg 2013;148(6):949–54.

18. Chan LS, Barakate MS, Havas TE. Free fat grafting in superficial parotid surgery to prevent Frey's syndrome and improve aesthetic outcome. J Laryngol Otol 2014;128(Suppl 1):S44–9.

19. Davis RE, Guida RA, Cook TA. Autologous free dermal fat graft. Reconstruction of facial contour defects. Arch Otolaryngol Head Neck Surg 1995;121(1): 95–100.

20. Honeybrook A, Athavale SM, Rangarajan SV, et al. Free dermal fat graft reconstruction of the head and neck: an alternate reconstructive option. Am J Otolaryngol 2017;38(3):291–6.

21. Militsakh ON, Sanderson JA, Lin D, et al. Rehabilitation of a parotidectomy patient–a systematic approach. Head Neck 2013;35(9):1349–61.

22. Lee YJ, Fischbein NJ, Megwalu U, et al. Radiographic surveillance of abdominal free fat graft in complex parotid pleomorphic adenomas: a case series. Heliyon 2020;6(5):e03894.

23. Cesteleyn L, Helman J, King S, et al. Temporoparietal fascia flaps and superficial musculoaponeurotic system plication in parotid surgery reduces Frey's syndrome. J Oral Maxillofac Surg 2002;60(11):1284–97, discussion 1297-1288.

24. Chen J, Lin F, Liu Z, et al. Pedicled temporalis muscle flap stuffing after a lateral temporal bone resection for treating mastoid osteoradionecrosis. Otolaryngol Head Neck Surg 2017;156(4):622–6.

25. Movassaghi K, Lewis M, Shahzad F, et al. Optimizing the aesthetic result of parotidectomy with a facelift incision and temporoparietal fascia flap. Plast Reconstr Surg Glob Open 2019;7(2):e2067.

26. Asal K, Koybasioglu A, Inal E, et al. Sternocleidomastoid muscle flap reconstruction during parotidectomy to prevent Frey's syndrome and facial contour deformity. Ear Nose Throat J 2005;84(3):173–6.

27. Gooden EA, Gullane PJ, Irish J, et al. Role of the sternocleidomastoid muscle flap preventing Frey's syndrome and maintaining facial contour following superficial parotidectomy. J Otolaryngol 2001;30(2):98–101.

28. Kerawala CJ, McAloney N, Stassen LF. Prospective randomised trial of the benefits of a sternocleidomastoid flap after superficial parotidectomy. Br J Oral Maxillofac Surg 2002;40(6):468–72.

29. Fee WE Jr, Tran LE. Functional outcome after total parotidectomy reconstruction. Laryngoscope 2004;114(2):223–6.

30. Bayon R, Davis AB. Submental flap for soft tissue reconstruction following radical parotidectomy. Otolaryngol Head Neck Surg 2019;160(6):1130–2.

31. Emerick KS, Herr MW, Lin DT, et al. Supraclavicular artery island flap for reconstruction of complex parotidectomy, lateral skull base, and total auriculectomy defects. JAMA Otolaryngol Head Neck Surg 2014;140(9):861–6.

32. Behan FC, Lo CH, Sizeland A, et al. Keystone island flap reconstruction of parotid defects. Plast Reconstr Surg 2012;130(1):36e–41e.

33. Cannady SB, Seth R, Fritz MA, et al. Total parotidectomy defect reconstruction using the buried free flap. Otolaryngol Head Neck Surg 2010;143(5): 637–43.
34. Thompson NJ, Roche JP, Schularick NM, et al. Reconstruction outcomes following lateral skull base resection. Otol Neurotol 2017;38(2):264–71.
35. Cigna E, Minni A, Barbaro M, et al. An experience on primary thinning and secondary debulking of anterolateral thigh flap in head and neck reconstruction. Eur Rev Med Pharmacol Sci 2012;16(8):1095–101.

Cosmetic Approaches to Parotidectomy

C. Alessandra Colaianni, MD[a], Jeremy D. Richmon, MD[b],*

KEYWORDS

- Parotidectomy • Cosmesis • Minimally invasive • Periauricular • Facelift
- Retroauricular • Endoscopic • Robotic

KEY POINTS

- The parotid gland lies in a cosmetically sensitive area. Over the past 80 years, since the modified Blair incision was introduced, several incisions designed to minimize scar visibility have been explored.
- Cosmetic incisional approaches to the parotid have included facelift/rhytidectomy with modifications, periauricular, and retroauricular incisions.
- Endoscopic and robotic approaches to the parotid recently have been described as means to minimize incision length and visibility.
- Research in this area is limited by small study size and incomplete outcomes data.
- More rigorous research is needed to ascertain the safety, cost-effectiveness, and feasibility of various cosmetic approaches to the parotid gland, particularly in cases of large, deep lobe, or malignant tumors.

INTRODUCTION/HISTORY/DEFINITIONS/BACKGROUND

Parotidectomy is a procedure performed primarily by otolaryngologists for both benign and malignant tumors of the parotid gland.[1] More than 3500 inpatient parotidectomies were performed in the United States in the year 2014.[2] Over the past half-century, increased attention has been paid to the cosmetic and patient-reported outcomes of surgeries of all varieties. This article reviews historical and cosmetically oriented approaches to parotid surgery.

When assessing the overall cosmetic impact of parotid surgery, several factors must be considered. First, maintaining full facial nerve function is of paramount importance. Even minor nerve injuries can result in subtle facial movement asymmetry, which may have a devastating psychosocial impact on the patient. For this reason, any approach to the parotid must maintain facial nerve identification and preservation

[a] Department of Otolaryngology, Vanderbilt University Medical Center, Medical Center East, South Tower, 1215 21st Avenue South, Suite 7209, Nashville, TN 37232, USA; [b] Department of Otolaryngology–Head and Neck Surgery, Harvard Medical School, Massachusetts Eye and Ear, 243 Charles Street, Boston, MA 02114, USA
* Corresponding author.
E-mail address: Jeremy_richmon@meei.harvard.edu

Otolaryngol Clin N Am 54 (2021) 583–591
https://doi.org/10.1016/j.otc.2021.02.010
0030-6665/21/© 2021 Elsevier Inc. All rights reserved.

oto.theclinics.com

as the absolute top priority. Second, maintaining soft tissue contour symmetry with the contralateral side is critical so as not to draw attention to the operated side. There are numerous methods of soft tissue volume restoration ranging from autologous tissue grafts, local muscle transfer, fat grafts, and free flaps, depending on the size of the parotid defect. Soft tissue reconstruction are discussed in Chapter 9. Finally, a noticeable and/or unsightly scar from parotid surgery can have a lifelong negative impact on a person's overall appearance. For this reason, there has been an evolution of approaches to make the incision less conspicuous.

The Blair incision, a preauricular approach to the parotid described by V.P. Blair in his seminal text, *Surgery and Diseases of the Mouth and Jaws*, offered the first widely publicized approach to parotid pathology. This text, published in 1912, was hailed in *The New England Journal of Medicine* (then the *Boston Medical and Surgical Journal*) as "the most satisfactory book dealing with this subdivision of surgery, that the reviewer has seen."[3] The Blair incision was a straight incision beginning in a preauricular crease and extending down the neck. The Blair incision was modified by Dr Hamilton Bailey[4] in 1941 (**Fig. 1**), adding a curve underneath the ear lobule as well as a cervical extension to permit improved exposure of the entire parotid gland. Bailey made this modification after noting that small tumors had a tendency to recur more often than larger tumors, hypothesizing that this was due to inadequate exposure and inadvertent tumor capsule violation.

As with any procedure in the head and neck, particularly for benign disease, cosmesis is an important consideration. Cosmesis was addressed directly by Bailey: "Contrary to what might be thought," he wrote, "Blair's incision gives an excellent cosmetic result." Bailey's modification notwithstanding, the search for ever more cosmetically appealing approaches to the parotid gland has continued in the 80 years following his 1941 publication. Of course, cosmesis always must be balanced against complications of parotidectomy, including facial nerve injury, sialocele, tumor spillage, tumor recurrence, and Frey syndrome. Novel approaches also must be evaluated for factors like equipment cost and operative time. As discussed, the tension Bailey observes in balancing cosmesis with adequate exposure has continued to the present day.

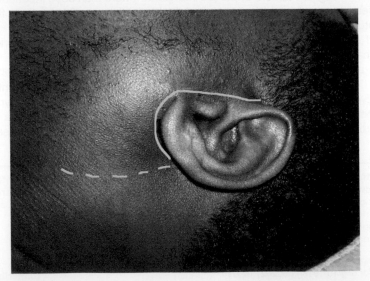

Fig. 1. Parotid Blair.

This article reviews various cosmetic approaches to the parotid gland and the available safety and outcomes data for each.

FACELIFT INCISION

The facelift or rhytidectomy-style incision (**Fig. 2**) first was described in reference to approaching parotid pathology by Appiani in 1967.[5,6] This incision originates at the superior root of the helix, follows the curve of the tragus, and curves superiorly around the lobule toward the mastoid, continuing in a postauricular crease to the occipital hairline and descending along the hairline. Many surgeons who use this technique for parotidectomy have since modified it, starting the incision in the preauricular crease rather than at the root of the helix and limiting the descending limb as needed. Perhaps due to its longstanding use, many studies specifically have addressed its safety and utility compared with the modified Blair incision. Grover and D'Souza[7] published the most comprehensive systematic review on the facelift approach for parotidectomy, reviewing studies published between 1960 and 2011, which included 11 studies with a total of 628 patients, for both benign and malignant pathology in both superficial and deep locations. They found no significant difference in operative time or complication rate between the facelift incision and the modified Blair incision. They also found that aesthetic outcomes pertaining to the postoperative scar favored the facelift incision. Noted limitations of the facelift incision in this systematic review included anterior exposure, use in obese patients, and restraint by fresh trainees.

RETROAURICULAR HAIRLINE INCISION

The retroauricular hairline incision as an approach to parotidectomy first was described formally in the literature in 2009. At that time, the retroauricular incision was limited to extracapsular dissection without facial nerve dissection, in mobile tumors located in the inferior superficial portion of the gland.[8] This incision extends upward from the postauricular sulcus, then curves downward, extending along the hairline (**Fig. 3**) (ie, similar to the facelift incision with the absence of the preauricular

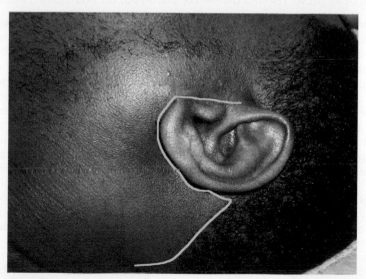

Fig. 2. Parotid facelift.

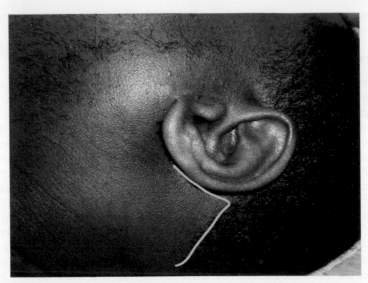

Fig. 3. Parotid retroauricular hairline.

component). In 2014, Kim and colleagues reported on 73 patients who underwent partial superficial parotidectomy rather than extracapsular dissection via this approach for previously untreated benign tumors, comparing them with patients undergoing facelift and modified Blair incisions.[9] Patients with tumors directly anterior to the external auditory canal were excluded. The Kim group reported no difference in operative time, location of tumor, size of tumor, occurrence of temporary or permanent facial nerve paralysis, or development of Frey syndrome. They did include tumors of the deep lobe of the parotid in their analysis. The retroauricular incision has also been used in conjunction with robotic or endoscopic approaches to the parotid.[10–12]

PERIAURICULAR (ALSO TERMED U-SHAPED, V-SHAPED, OR POSTAURAL) INCISION

The periauricular incision for parotid surgery is favored by the senior author in his approach to both benign and low-grade malignant parotid pathologies not requiring a concomitant neck dissection. The incision begins in the pretragal crease (retrotragal if no crease is present in young women), is carried around the earlobe, and extends into the postauricular crease. It differs from the facelift incision in that it does not continue superiorly to the postauricular hairline and does not have a descending limb down the hairline. The incision and its application to a patient with a 5-cm pleomorphic adenoma can be viewed in **Fig. 4**. Data on the periauricular incision are limited: it has been described previously in small studies limited by small numbers of patients and narrow outcomes data. Petroianu[13] and Yuen[14] reported a series of 41 and 69 patients respectively but did not include facial nerve outcomes. Wu and colleagues[15] reported 16 consecutive periauricular approaches to benign tumors of the parotid gland, with 2 patients suffering temporary facial nerve paralysis; however, this study was limited by the small number of patients reported. The authors' retrospective analysis of 97 patients undergoing parotidectomy showed no significant difference in postoperative complications, facial nerve outcomes, length of stay, or operative time.[16] The authors report a small but significant difference in tumor size, with tumors an average of 2.1 cm in periauricular patients compared with 2.6 cm in modified Blair or facelift patients.

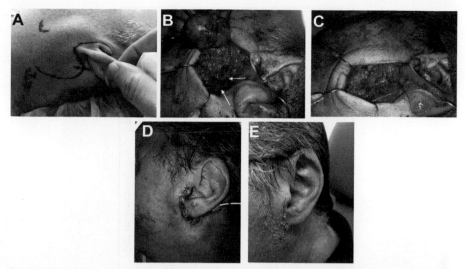

Fig. 4. (*A*) Periauricular and modified Blair incision drawn on a preoperative patient. The crossed line indicates where the periauricular incision stops. (*B*) Facial nerve identification and tumor mobilization. The white arrow denotes the great auricular nerve. The yellow arrow denotes the main trunk of the facial nerve. (*C*) Tumor removal. (*D*) Immediate postoperative appearance. (*E*) Appearance of incision after drain removal.

ENDOSCOPIC-ASSISTED APPROACH

An endoscopic-assisted approach to parotidectomy has been described by 2 separate groups, with the aim of improving cosmesis over a traditional parotidectomy incision. These groups used the previously described retroauricular hairline incision with custom-made retractors to elevate skin flaps and endoscopic harmonic scalpels for tissue dissection. Chen and colleagues[10] described 30 patients who underwent parotidectomy for benign pathology via a 4-cm to 5.5-cm curved retroauricular incision, compared with an age-matched, sex-matched, and tumor volume–matched control group who underwent conventional parotidectomy They reported statistically significant shorter incision lengths, bleeding volume, and operative times with the endoscopic group as well as improved subjective satisfaction with the scar. Li and colleagues[11] described 15 patients who underwent parotidectomy for benign or low-grade malignant pathology via a 4-cm retroauricular incision with endoscopic assistance; they compared these patients to 57 patients who underwent a modified Blair incision. They reported no significant difference in perioperative indicators, such as blood loss, operation time, tumor diameter, or hospital stay. They also reported that the aesthetic satisfaction based on patient survey data favored the endoscopic group.

ROBOT-ASSISTED APPROACH

One group has reported a novel robot-assisted approach to parotidectomy for improved cosmetic outcomes. Park and colleagues[12] recently reported a series of 53 patients undergoing da Vinci Xi (Intuitive, Sunnyvale CA) robot–assisted parotidectomy for benign or malignant pathology, with or without concomitant robot-assisted neck dissection. All patients had a retroauricular incision extending down the hairline. The approach required 2 assistants for retraction during flap elevation, during which

Table 1
Comparison of minimally invasive approaches to parotidectomy

Approach	Year Introduced	Level of Evidence	Surgical Time	Relative Contraindications	Complication Rates	Need for Special Equipment	Additional Cost
Facelift	1967	II (systematic review)	No difference to standard approaches	Tumors requiring significant anterior exposure, obese patients	No difference to standard approaches	No	None
Retroauricular	2009	III	No difference to standard approaches	Malignant tumors, tumors directly anterior to external auditory canal	No difference to standard approaches	No	None
Periauricular	2016	III	No difference to standard approaches	Patients requiring concomitant neck dissection	No difference to standard approaches	No	None
Endoscopic-assisted	2014	III	No difference to standard approaches	Deep lobe tumors, tumors without clear borders	No difference to standard approaches	Yes	Yes
Robot-assisted	2020	IV	Not measured	None reported	Not measured	Yes	Yes

the robot was docked and only robotic instruments were used. The number of trocars used was not reported. The group reported temporary facial paralysis in 3 cases and an average console time of between 100 minutes and 200 minutes, which stabilized at 100 minutes after the first 5 cases. This article did not specifically compare outcomes from robot-assisted parotidectomy to traditional incisional approaches.

In the authors' opinion, these technology-assisted approaches have the same resultant scar as the periauricular approach without any notable benefit (**Table 1**). The authors, therefore, find it hard to justify the additional equipment, operative time, and overall cost of these technology-assisted approaches.

DISCUSSION

Literature from other areas of head and neck surgery, including endocrine surgery, suggest that a visible scar on a patient's neck or face can have a significant impact on self-perception and quality of life, even years after their initial operation.[17,18] This can lead to functional impairment and significant psychosocial burden.[19] It follows that the impact of scars on the face and neck after parotidectomy, if visually unappealing, can have a negative impact on patients' quality of life.[20] Cosmetically oriented, minimal, or exceptionally well-hidden scars are rated more favorably by patients than modified Blair incisions in several studies.[21,22]

Several approaches to the parotid that emphasize cosmesis have been described over the past 80 years, including the facelift or rhytidectomy-style incision, retroauricular hairline incisions, and periauricular/U-shaped/V-shaped/postaural incisions. Data on the safety and efficacy of these approaches are limited. The quality of the studies varies. In general, they appear to be safe for the majority of parotid pathologies. Caution should be taken, however, for extended parotid approaches, such as the deep lobe, or in a suspected malignancy when a concomitant neck dissection may be required. Further research is needed to delineate appropriate and safe usage of each approach. Finally, validated quality-of-life instruments should be used to assess the patients' perspectives for each procedure.

SUMMARY

The parotid gland is located in a cosmetically sensitive area. Given cultural emphasis on cosmesis, using minimally invasive or hidden incisions, when appropriate, can significantly improve patient satisfaction and quality of life following surgery. Facelift-style incisions have been used since the late 1960s to approach parotid pathology. Several alternative incisions, including technology-assisted approaches, also have been described in the literature. To that end, the existing data regarding several historical and emerging cosmetic approaches to the parotid gland are described.

CLINICS CARE POINTS

- The parotid gland lies in a cosmetically sensitive area. Over the past 80 years, less conspicuous incision options have been explored.

- Cosmetic incisional approaches to the parotid have included modified Blair, facelift/ rhytidectomy with modifications, periauricular, and retroauricular incisions.

- Endoscopic and robotic approaches to the parotid recently have been described as means to minimize incision length and visibility.

- Research in this area is limited by small study size and incomplete outcomes data.
- More rigorous research is needed to ascertain the safety, cost-effectiveness, and feasibility of various cosmetic approaches to the parotid gland, particularly in cases of large, deep lobe, or malignant tumors.

DISCLOSURE

The authors have no disclosures to report.

REFERENCES

1. Larian B. Parotidectomy for benign parotid tumors. Otolaryngol Clin North Am 2016;49(2):395–413.
2. Sethi RKV, Deschler EG. National trends in inpatient parotidectomy: a fourteen-year retrospective analysis. Am J Otolaryngol 2018;39:553–7.
3. Reviewed in Boston Med Surg J, 1913;169–95.
4. Bailey H. The treatment of tumours of the parotid gland with special reference to total parotidectomy. Br J Surg 1941;(111):337–46.
5. Appiani E. Abordage para la parotidectomia y transplante muscular. Prensa Med Argent 1967;52:124.
6. Appiani E, Delfino MC. Plastic incisions for facial and neck tumors. Ann Plast Surg 1984;13(4):335–52.
7. Grover N, D'Souza A. Facelift approach for parotidectomy: an evolving aesthetic technique. Otolaryngol Head Neck Surg 2013;148($):548–56.
8. Roh JL. Extracapsular dissection of benign parotid tumors using a retroauricular hairline incision approach. Am J Surg 2009;197:e53–6.
9. Kim DY, Park GC, Cho YW, et al. Partial superficial parotidectomy via retroauricular hairline incision. Clin Exp Otorhinolaryngol 2014;7(2):119–22.
10. Chen J, Chen W, Zhang J, et al. Modified Endoscope-Assisted Partial-Superficial Parotidectomy through a retroauricular incision. ORL J Otorhinolaryngol Relat Spec 2014;76(3):121–6.
11. Li T, Liu Y, Wang Q, et al. Parotidectomy by an endoscopic-assisted postauricular groove approach. Head Neck 2019;41:2851–9.
12. Park YM, Kim DH, Kang MS, et al. Real impact of surgical robotic system for precision surgery of parotidectomy: retroauricular parotidectomy using da Vinci surgical system. Gland Surg 2020;9(2):183–91.
13. Petroianu A. Parotidectomy by periauricular incision. Otolaryngol Head Neck Surg 2012;146(2):247–9.
14. Yuen AP. Small access postaural parotidectomy: an analysis of techniques, feasibility and safety. Eur Arch Otorhinolaryngol 2016;273(*7):1879–83.
15. Wu PA, Liang WY, Lu ZQ, et al. Functional modified periauricular incision in parotidectomy. Lin Chung Er Bi Yan Hou Tou Jing Wai Ke Za Zhi 2017;31(13):995–7.
16. Colaianni CA, Feng AL, Richmon JR. Partial parotidectomy via periauricular incision: retrospective cohort study and comparative analysis to alternative incisional approaches. Head Neck 2020. https://doi.org/10.1002/hed.26542.
17. Linos D, Christodoulou S, Kutsou V, et al. Health-related quality of life and cosmesis after thyroidectomy: long-term outcomes. World J Surg 2020;44(1):134–41.
18. Choi Y, Lee JH, Kim YH, et al. Impact of postthyroidectomy scar on the quality of life of thyroid cancer patients. Ann Dermatol 2014;26:693–9.

19. Arora A, Swords C, Garas G, et al. The perception of scar cosmesis following thyroid and parathyroid surgery: A prospective cohort study. Int J Surg 2016;25: 38–43.
20. Ciuman RR, Oels W, Jaussi R, et al. Outcome, general, and symptom-specific quality of life after various types of parotid resection. Laryngoscope 2012; 122(6):1254–61.
21. Lorenz KJ, Behringer PA, Hocherl D, et al. Improving the quality of life of parotid surgery patients through a modified facelift incision and great auricular nerve preservation. GMS Interdiscip Plast Reconstr Surg DGPW 2013;(2):1–7.
22. Roh JL, Kim HS, Park CI. Randomized clinical trial comparing partial parotidectomy versus superficial or total parotidectomy. Br J Surg 2007;94:1081–7.

Observation Rather than Surgery for Benign Parotid Tumors: Why, When, and How

Barak Ringel, MD, Dennis Kraus, MD*

KEYWORDS

- Benign parotid lesions • Parotidectomy • Observation • Salivary gland
- Malignant transformation

KEY POINTS

- Most benign parotid lesions require surgical excision.
- Surgery provides a histologic definition of the lesion and prevents lesion enlargement and malignant transformation.
- Parotidectomy and anesthesia-related morbidities are sometimes inevitable.
- There are no guidelines or published literature that recommend when observation for a benign parotid lesion is superior to surgical excision.
- When considering observation, many factors should be taken into account, including presumed histology, risk of malignant transformation, tumor size, the involvement of vital structures, patient's age, medical comorbidities, surgical and anesthesia-related morbidity, and the patient's will.

INTRODUCTION

A well-known aphorism in medicine states that good surgeons know how to operate, better ones know when to operate, and the most experienced surgeons know when not to operate. The morbidity related to any surgery, starting from the time of incising the skin, must be weighed against the benefits of treatment. Hence surgeons confronted with benign parotid lesions should have the courage of their convictions and follow the dictate of *primum non nocere*. The treatment should be based on many factors, and it takes wisdom, experience, strength, and fortitude to make the right decision and commit to these principles.

In other regions of the head and neck, such as the larynx, the concept of organ preservation is well established.[1–3] Attempts to define functional interoperability has been made for the oral cavity and oropharynx,[4]

The Department of Otolaryngology-Head & Neck Surgery, Lenox Hill Hospital / Northwell Health, 130 East 77th Street - Black Hall 10th Floor, New York, NY 10075, USA
* Corresponding author.
E-mail address: dkraus@northwell.edu

Otolaryngol Clin N Am 54 (2021) 593–604
https://doi.org/10.1016/j.otc.2021.02.004
0030-6665/21/© 2021 Elsevier Inc. All rights reserved.

oto.theclinics.com

The inevitable incidence of general morbidity from surgery and anesthesia, and specifically complications arising from salivary gland surgery, make it challenging to assess when it is appropriate to observe a likely benign salivary gland lesion. There is no sound evidence in the literature dealing with the question of when to avoid surgical excision of a parotid lesion. Identifying the confluence of disease factors and patient characteristics that together indicate that surgery should be avoided is complex. This article addresses the question and discusses the circumstances in which observation is considered superior to surgical treatment of benign parotid lesions.

DISCUSSION

There are two leading theories accounting for the origin of salivary gland neoplasms. The multicenter theory posits that each type of neoplasm originates from a distinctive cell type within the salivary gland unit, whereas the bicellular reserve cell theory assumes that all types of salivary neoplasm originate from basal cells of either the excretory or the intercalated duct.[5–9]

Besides exposure to irradiation, there are no known risk factors for salivary gland neoplasms or salivary gland malignancies. The association of specific genetic abnormalities with other environmental factors (viruses, diet, occupational exposure) may lead to an increased risk of developing salivary gland tumors, but are not decisive factors in making a decision.[10–12] Most benign parotid lesions need to be excised. There is abundant literature on reasons for the excision of these lesions, motivated primarily by the need to have definitive histologic confirmation, prevention of further growth and avoidance of the rare event of malignant transformation.[13–16] Some patients demand surgical excision because of cosmetic impairment or fear of malignancy.

This article discusses the factors and circumstances that should be taken into account when considering observation versus surgical treatment.

History

The lesion should be well characterized, as should the patient's medical and surgical history. History in part provides guidelines for appropriate treatment. Inflammation, infection, or outflow obstruction might present as a new parotid lump or enlargement and should be ruled out. Local pain, rapid growth, and facial nerve weakness may suggest that the lesion is malignant. Other features include a history of skin lesions, neck adenopathy, and constitutional complaints. Aside from previous irradiation exposure, there are no proven risk factors for the development of benign and malignant salivary gland lesions.[10–12,17]

Physical Examination

The approach to parotid lesions should follow the procedure for any other neck lump. The size, consistency, mobility, and adherence to surrounding structures, such as the skin, or underlying structures should be identified. The neck should be carefully examined to identify lymphadenopathy or other masses. The function of the facial nerve and other cranial nerve should be assessed. Signs of infection should be carefully sought, and signs of inflammation or impacted stones. The other salivary glands should be assessed to rule out concomitant lesions. The face and scalp should be assessed to identify skin lesions that might represent a skin primary. The oropharynx should be assessed for asymmetricity or bulges to rule out parapharyngeal involvement.

Imaging

Imaging should be used routinely for the evaluation of parotid lesions because it can contribute essential information to the treatment decision-making process. Imaging can show the tumor location within the gland; its relationship to the facial nerve or other neurovascular structures; and its extent into the parapharynx, skull base, or the skin. Several specific characteristics can help differentiate malignant from benign entities, including the contour of the lesion, its content, its infiltration pattern, or neck lymph node involvement, all of which can help define the nature of the lesion.[18,19]

MRI provides superior imaging of the parotid fat and soft tissue content. The enhancement of certain pathologies is pathognomonic for lesions, such as pleomorphic adenoma or Warthin tumor. Although rare, certain pathologies, such as lipoma, vascular malformations, cysts, or other congenital masses, are well-visualized by MRI. Computed tomography (CT) can also show the anatomy of the gland and the tumor and the skeletal structure of the adjacent skull base. It is more accessible but provides less definition than MRI for soft tissue architecture and planes.[20–24]

Ultrasonography is widely available, inexpensive, noninvasive, and has no associated complications. It can direct accurate fine-needle aspiration (FNA) biopsy, which can help define some salivary gland pathologies and distinguish solid from cystic or vascular malformations (by using Doppler when available).[25–28] PET/CT is not a reliable tool for defining benign or malignant lesions because salivary gland lesions have different fluorodeoxyglucose avidity, which makes it impossible to differentiate benign from malignant origins. PET/CT is useful in known malignancies in excluding nodal or distant metastatic disease.[29–33] Some tumors show increased predilection for technetium-99m pertechnetate, and thus, it may serve to distinguish between tumors, such as Warthin and oncocytoma, which often enhance on a radionucleotide scan, to those that do not, such as pleomorphic adenoma.[34]

Biopsy

FNA is the best established technique for salivary gland lesion evaluation. Its sensitivity is 78%, with a specificity of 98% in distinguishing malignant from benign parotid disease. In some instances, it is still difficult to distinguish benign from malignant pathologies because certain benign-malignant pathologies are similar, which leads to a diagnostic challenge.[35–37] The senior author has adopted FNA/core needle biopsy as a routine method for evaluation and treatment planning. It serves to avoid unnecessary surgery for inflammatory etiologies, lymphomas, or other pathologies that do not require complete excision. Core needle biopsy can improve diagnostic accuracy, but studies have reported higher likelihoods of hematoma formation and tumor seeding. Other studies have found FNA to be safer than core needle biopsy.[38] The Milan system for reporting salivary gland cytopathology can lead to better communication between the pathology team and the surgeon. It categorizes the likelihood of malignancy, and makes it possible to avoid surgery in specific cases classified as Milan II (10% of all malignancies) and IV-benign (<5% risk of malignancy) (**Table 1**).[39–41]

Risks of Parotidectomy

Facial paralysis, either temporary or permanent, is devastating for the patient, and can affect not only quality of life and appearance, but can also lead to significant functional disabilities, which can result in severe eye complications and less commonly, swallowing abnormalities. Complications, such as sialocele, sensory deficit, Frey syndrome, scar formation, and hematoma formation, are even more common (**Table 2**). Parotidectomy should be considered with appropriate consideration of these possible risks. Although most lesions require surgery, some do not, and the risks of surgery must be carefully weighed against its benefits and thoroughly discussed with the patient. The surgeon must have the required skills, experience, equipment, and setup to minimize complications.[42–47]

Table 1
The Milan system for reporting salivary gland cytopathology: implied risks of malignancy and recommended clinical management

Diagnostic Category	Risk of Malignancy (%)	Management
I. Nondiagnostic	25	Clinical and radiologic correlation/repeat fine-needle aspiration cytology
II. Nonneoplastic	10	Clinical follow-up and radiologic correlation
III. Atypia of undetermined significance	20	Repeat fine-needle aspiration cytology or surgery
IV. Neoplasm		
Neoplasm: benign	<5	Surgery or clinical follow-up
Neoplasm: salivary gland neoplasm of uncertain malignant potential	35	Surgery
V. Suspicious for malignancy	60	Surgery
VI. Malignant	90	Surgery

Risks of Anesthesia and Postoperative Recovery

All surgical procedures involve possible significant anesthesia-related risks. There are many adverse perioperative and postoperative events that should be taken into account, including the risk of respiratory, cardiovascular, cerebrovascular events, hematologic incidents, and others that may lead to permanent disabilities and even death. Cognitive status should be well assessed as for any other surgical procedure. Advanced dementia should prompt discussion of the benefits and burden of surgical and nonsurgical management with the family or guardians. Life expectancy is another factor that should be taken into account, although advanced age by itself may not preclude an elective surgery with acceptable mortality risk. The risks of anesthesia should be considered for all patients, and in particular for those with comorbidities, advanced age, or increased body mass index. Some authors even suggested that parotidectomy

Table 2
Parotidectomy complication rates

Complication	Rate (%)
Temporary facial weakness	10–40
Permanent facial weakness	0–15
Greater auricular nerve anesthesia	0–25
Postoperative hematoma	0–7
Frey syndrome	5–80
Salivary fistula	0–10
Sialocele	0–15
Infection	0–5
Sensory deficit	0–20
Seroma	0–10
Keloid formation	0–1

performed under local anesthesia may be a reasonable option for elderly patients. A recent study using a decision analytical Markov model suggested that observation may be favorable for patients older than 70 years with pleomorphic adenoma.[48–55] The American College of Surgeons National Surgical Improvement Program has developed a surgical risk calculator, which is accessed as an online tool (**Fig. 1**). The risk of significant negative outcomes, ranging from minor complications to severe adverse events, such as disability or death, must be carefully considered against the presumed pathology and need for surgery.[56–58]

Pathology

Although the parotid is the most common gland affected by tumors compared with other salivary glands, studies have shown that malignancy rate of parotid lesions is the lowest (15%) of all.[12,59–61] The goals of parotidectomy for benign histology is defining the pathology, avoiding growth, and preventing malignant transformation. In cases where a clear diagnosis is made by biopsy and imaging, surgery may be a consideration. The most common benign parotid lesions are pleomorphic adenoma (80%–90% of cases) and Warthin tumor (7%–10%). Other inflammatory, congenital lesions, and other etiologies are listed in **Table 3**.[62,63]

Benign tumors

Pleomorphic adenoma (benign mixed tumor) manifests as a slow-growing, painless mass, which may be present for years. Lesion location often determines its symptoms,

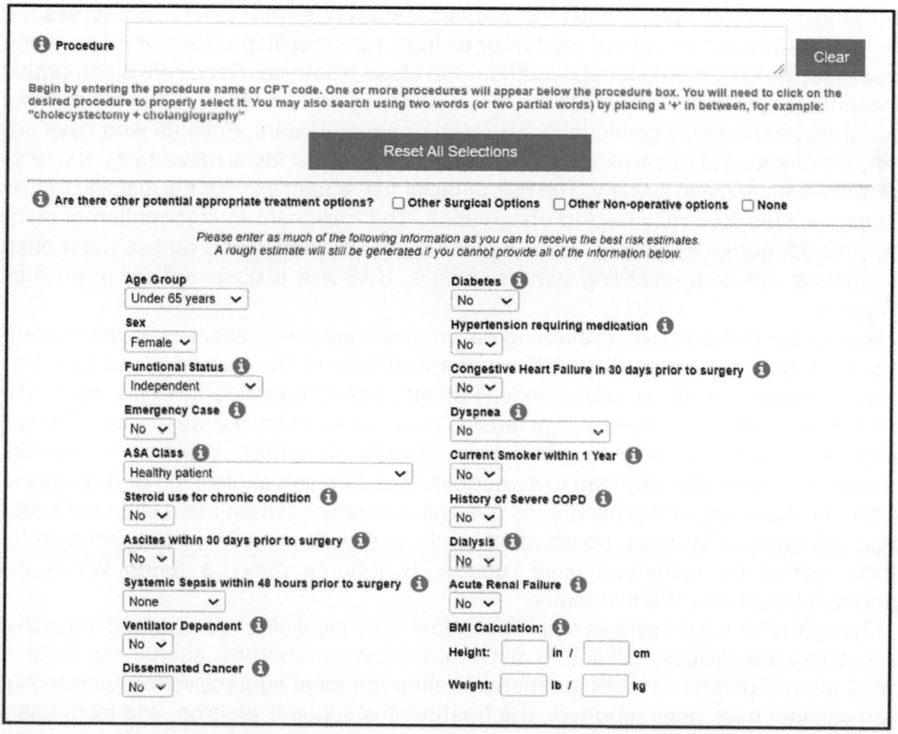

Fig. 1. The American College of Surgeons National Surgical Improvement Program (ASCS-NSQIP) surgical risk calculator.[56] BMI, body mass index; COPD, chronic obstructive pulmonary disease.

Table 3 World Health Organization histology classification of salivary gland lesions	
Benign tumors	Pleomorphic adenoma
	Warthin tumor
	Myoepithelioma
	Basal cell adenoma
	Oncocytoma
	Lymphadenoma
	Cystadenoma
	Sialadenoma papilliform
	Ductal papillomas
	Sebaceous adenoma
	Canalicular adenoma and other ductal adenomas
Nonneoplastic epithelial lesions	Sclerosing polycystic adenosis
	Nodular oncocytic hyperplasia
	Lymphoepithelial sialadenitis
	Intercalated duct hyperplasia
Benign soft tissue lesions	Hemangioma
	Lipoma/sialolipoma
	Nodular fasciitis

such as facial nerve weakness or retrotonsillar budge when the deep lobe is involved. The recommended treatment of pleomorphic adenomas is surgical excision with a surrounding cuff of normal tissue to prevent recurrence from failure to address the pseudopod-like extensions of the tumor or from tumor spillage. Nevertheless, some cases may be considered for observation with close follow-up. Recurrent pleomorphic adenoma is rare, but when it occurs, it is a challenging problem. Frequently multiple foci of recurrence may continue to manifest for several years. Patients who have undergone previous surgical excision are at increased risk for facial nerve injury and rerecurrence with revision surgery. The risk of facial nerve paralysis, or the inability to fully excise multiple foci, may lead to observation. The malignant transformation of pleomorphic adenoma is rare (but when it occurs can be deadly) and occurs most often in patients with long-standing tumors, with a 10% risk if observed for more than 15 years.

Warthin tumors (papillary cystadenoma lymphomatosum) present as an asymptomatic, slow-growing mass often in the superficial lobe of the parotid gland that may affect the patient's facial appearance. Patients can experience swelling, pain, and other inflammatory changes. Large lesions may cause cosmetic deformity, whereas large resections may lead to significant cosmetic deformity. Infection or the rare case of multicentricity may lead to inadequate excision and explain tumor recurrence. Although treatment of Warthin tumor is surgical excision, when there is sound histologic evidence of Warthin, observation could suffice for small, indistinguishable lesions. Based on numerous case reports, lymphoma may be found within the lymphoid tissue of a Warthin tumor.

Myoepitheliomas present as a painless, slow-growing well-circumscribed mass that sometimes are clinically difficult to distinguish from pleomorphic adenomas. Most of these tumors behave in a benign manner, although local aggressiveness and malignant variants have been reported. The treatment is surgical excision, and incomplete excision is associated with recurrence.

Basal cell adenoma (monomorphic adenoma) presents as a slow-growing, mobile, asymptomatic mass. Basal cell adenoma may be difficult to distinguish from the solid variant of adenoid cystic carcinoma or other malignancies; hence the treatment is surgical excision with a cuff of normal surrounding tissue.

Oncocytoma presents as painless, slowly enlarging tumors that may mimic some types of malignant salivary tumors with oncocytic components, such as mucoepidermoid carcinoma, adenoid cystic carcinoma and adenocarcinoma, or metastases from renal cell or thyroid carcinoma. It has a destructive potential; thus, the treatment is surgical excision.

Cystadenoma is a rare benign neoplasm, slow growing painless, sometimes presenting as a multicystic mass. It may be confused with mucocele. Surgical excision and conservative observation may be appropriate.

Nonneoplastic epithelial lesions

Sclerosing polycystic adenosis has a histologic resemblance to fibrocystic changes of the breast. This entity presents as a slow-growing mass, and recurrence occurs in 15% of cases after surgical excision. Nodular oncocytic hyperplasia is characterized by multiple nodular proliferations, that is associated with an human papillomavirus infection. Treatment is surgical excision; however, when there is a confirmed cytologic diagnosis, observation may be considered.

Lymphoepithelial sialadenitis (Mikulicz syndrome) is considered a benign autoimmune lesion, which may be a cardinal component of Sjögren syndrome, but also has some association to AIDS. It presents as a painless, unilateral/bilateral parotid mass. It has a risk of transformation to MALT lymphoma. Observation is adequate, with good response to steroid treatment or needle aspiration.

IgG4-related salivary gland disease (chronic sclerosing sialadenitis, Kuttner tumor, Mikulicz disease) presents as a hard swelling that is unilateral or bilateral and indistinguishable from a tumor. This disease process belongs to the spectrum of IgG4-related sclerosing disease. Some patients have associated autoimmune disease. The serum levels of IgG, IgG4, and IgG4/IgG ratio are typically elevated. Treatment with steroids is associated with an excellent response.

Congenital lesions

Hemangiomas of the parotid area usually present with a rapid growth phase (around the age of 1–12 months), followed by gradual involution by 9 years. Patients are usually asymptomatic, whereas the overlying skin may be normal, or may be involved in the disease. In cases of extremely large lesions, it may cause bleeding, heart failure, and even death. Treatment initially should consist of the nonselective β-blocker (propranolol) with excellent success rates, but other treatment options include steroids, interferon, endovascular sclerotherapy, laser therapy, and surgical excision.

Lipoadenoma (sialolipoma) is defined as a slowly growing mass that consists of lipomatous and epithelial components in the parotid. Complete excision is curative.

THE LONG-TERM EVIDENCE OF OBSERVATION STRATEGIES
Benign to Malignant Tumor Transformation

As noted, the 15-year 9.5% malignant transformation leads to the decisive surgical excision for malignant potential pleomorphic adenoma.[64–68] Other benign lesions have no proved potential for malignant transformation.

Recurrent Tumors

Some tumor recurrences pose a huge problem because of the multifocal involvement and seeding of the surgical field that might occur during surgical excision. In such cases, careful consideration should be given to the efficacy of surgery versus observation or irradiation therapy. The follow-up should involve an annual MRI and consideration of tumor location; size; enlargement rate; and involvement of the facial nerve, skin, parapharyngeal space, and so forth. The timing of reoperation is another important factor to take into account with respect to the postoperative inflammatory response, soft tissue adhesion, and scar tissue formation.[69,70]

Unresectable Tumors

Rarely, tumors with evidence of benign histology are unresectable because of their size, location, infiltration, or the involvement of adjacent structures. The credo of *primum non nocera* dictates the obligation to avoid causing damage to function or putting the patient at risk. In these cases, observation might be safer than surgery. This includes cases where the facial nerve is surrounded by the tumor, there is involvement of the deep parotid lobe, and extension to the parapharyngeal space or other circumstances that can damage adjacent neurovascular structures.

SUMMARY

The minority of benign parotid lesions meet the criteria for observation rather than surgical excision. There are no definite guidelines or supporting literature that define cases that require observation. The treating surgeon must include in his or her basket of considerations factors that include tumor and patient characteristics when weighting observation as the chosen modality. When observation is chosen, the patient should be followed frequently and cautiously, and the surgeon should be prepared to change strategy to surgical excision if in doubt.

CLINICS CARE POINTS

- Most patients require surgical excision of benign and malignant tumors.
- The decision to observe a parotid tumor most commonly is predicated on medical comorbidities and the risk of anesthesia complications.
- A minority of the parotid lesions with specific proved appropriate benign histology allow close observation and refrain from surgical excision.
- In elderly patients, surgical risks of facial nerve injury and other morbidities may outweigh the tumor-associated morbidity and mortality risk.
- Recurrent tumors constitute a problem because of scar tissue formation, adhesions, and multicentricity, and therefore pose an increased risk of damage to vital neurovascular structures when reoperated.

CONFLICT OF INTEREST DISCLOSURES

The authors have no funding, financial relationships, or conflicts of interest to disclose.

REFERENCES

1. Forastiere AA, Goepfert H, Maor M, et al. Concurrent chemotherapy and radiotherapy for organ preservation in advanced laryngeal cancer. N Engl J Med 2003;349(22):2091–8.
2. Wolf GT, Fisher SG, Hong WK, et al. Induction chemotherapy plus radiation compared with surgery plus radiation in patients with advanced laryngeal cancer. N Engl J Med 1991;324(24):1685–90.

3. Forastiere AA, Zhang Q, Weber RS, et al. Long-term results of RTOG 91-11: a comparison of three nonsurgical treatment strategies to preserve the larynx in patients with locally advanced larynx cancer. J Clin Oncol 2013;31(7):845–52.

4. Kreeft A, Tan IB, Van Den Brekel MWM, et al. The surgical dilemma of "functional inoperability" in oral and oropharyngeal cancer: current consensus on operability with regard to functional results. Clin Otolaryngol 2009;34(2):140–6.

5. Dardick I, Byard RW, Carnegie JA. A review of the proliferative capacity of major salivary glands and the relationship to current concepts of neoplasia in salivary glands. Oral Surg Oral Med Oral Pathol 1990;69(1):53–67.

6. Redman RS. Myoepithelium of salivary glands. Microsc Res Tech 1994;27(1): 25–45.

7. Dardick I, Burford-Mason AP. Current status of histogenetic and morphogenetic concepts of salivary gland tumorigenesis. Crit Rev Oral Biol Med 1994;4(5): 639–77.

8. Denny PC, Ball WD, Redman RS. Salivary glands: a paradigm for diversity of gland development. Crit Rev Oral Biol Med 1997;8(1):51–75.

9. Batsakis JG, Regezi JA, Luna MA, et al. Histogenesis of salivary gland neoplasms: a postulate with prognostic implications. J Laryngol Otol 1989;103(10): 939–44.

10. Spitz MR, Tilley BC, Batsakis JG, et al. Risk factors for major salivary gland carcinoma. A case-comparison study. Cancer 1984;54(9):1854–9.

11. Horn-Ross PL, Ljung BM, Morrow M. Environmental factors and the risk of salivary gland cancer. Epidemiology 1997;8(4):414–9.

12. Spiro RH. Salivary neoplasms: overview of a 35-year experience with 2,807 patients. Head Neck Surg 1986;8(3):177–84.

13. Quer M, Vander Poorten V, Takes RP, et al. Surgical options in benign parotid tumors: a proposal for classification. Eur Arch Otorhinolaryngol 2017;274(11): 3825–36.

14. Sood S, McGurk M, Vaz F. Management of salivary gland tumours: United Kingdom National Multidisciplinary Guidelines. J Laryngol Otol 2016;130(S2): S142–9.

15. Adelstein DJ, Koyfman SA, El-Naggar AK, et al. Biology and management of salivary gland cancers. Semin Radiat Oncol 2012;22(3):245–53.

16. Cheuk W, Chan JKC. Advances in salivary gland pathology. Histopathology 2007; 51(1):1–20.

17. Kane WJ, McCaffrey TV, Olsen KD, et al. Primary parotid malignancies: a clinical and pathologic review. Arch Otolaryngol Head Neck Surg 1991;117(3):307–15.

18. Silvers AR, Som PM. Salivary glands. Radiol Clin North Am 1998;36(5):941–66, vi.

19. Yousem DM, Kraut MA, Chalian AA. Major salivary gland imaging. Radiology 2000;216(1):19–29.

20. Choi DS, Na DG, Byun HS, et al. Salivary gland tumors: evaluation with two-phase helical CT. Radiology 2000;214(1):231–6.

21. Casselman JW, Mancuso AA. Major salivary gland masses: comparison of MR imaging and CT. Radiology 1987;165(1):183–9.

22. Thoeny HC. Imaging of salivary gland tumors. Cancer Imaging 2007;7(1):52–62.

23. Freling NJ, Molenaar WM, Vermey A, et al. Malignant parotid tumors: clinical use of MR imaging and histologic correlation. Radiology 1992;185(3):691–6.

24. Christe A, Waldherr C, Hallett R, et al. MR imaging of parotid tumors: typical lesion characteristics in MR imaging improve discrimination between benign and malignant disease. AJNR Am J Neuroradiol 2011;32(7):1202–7.

25. Bozzato A, Zenk J, Greess H, et al. Potential of ultrasound diagnosis for parotid tumors: analysis of qualitative and quantitative parameters. Otolaryngol Head Neck Surg 2007;137(4):642–6.
26. Bialek EJ, Jakubowski W, Zajkowski P, Szopinski KT, Osmolski A. US of the major salivary glands: anatomy and spatial relationships, pathologic conditions, and pitfalls. Radiogr a Rev Publ Radiol Soc North Am Inc 2006;26(3):745–63.
27. Yonetsu K, Ohki M, Kumazawa S, et al. Parotid tumors: differentiation of benign and malignant tumors with quantitative sonographic analyses. Ultrasound Med Biol 2004;30(5):567–74.
28. Brennan PA, Herd MK, Howlett DC, et al. Is ultrasound alone sufficient for imaging superficial lobe benign parotid tumours before surgery? Br J Oral Maxillofac Surg 2012;50(4):333–7.
29. Basu S, Houseni M, Alavi A. Significance of incidental fluorodeoxyglucose uptake in the parotid glands and its impact on patient management. Nucl Med Commun 2008;29(4):367–73.
30. Hadiprodjo D, Ryan T, Truong MT, et al. Parotid gland tumors: preliminary data for the value of FDG PET/CT diagnostic parameters. Am J Roentgenol 2012;198(2): 185–90.
31. Seo YL, Yoon DY, Baek S, et al. Incidental focal FDG uptake in the parotid glands on PET/CT in patients with head and neck malignancy. Eur Radiol 2015;25(1): 171–7.
32. Razfar A, Heron DE, Branstetter IVBF, et al. Positron emission tomography-computed tomography adds to the management of salivary gland malignancies. Laryngoscope 2010;120(4):734–8.
33. Makis W, Ciarallo A, Gotra A. Clinical significance of parotid gland incidentalomas on 18F-FDG PET/CT. Clin Imaging 2015;39(4):667–71.
34. Kikuchi M, Koyasu S, Shinohara S, et al. Preoperative diagnostic strategy for parotid gland tumors using diffusion-weighted MRI and technetium-99m pertechnetate scintigraphy: a prospective study. PLoS One 2016;11(2):1–17.
35. Howlett DC, Skelton E, Moody AB. Establishing an accurate diagnosis of a parotid lump: evaluation of the current biopsy methods - fine needle aspiration cytology, ultrasound-guided core biopsy, and intraoperative frozen section. Br J Oral Maxillofac Surg 2015;53(7):580–3.
36. Liu H, Ljungren C, Lin F, et al. Analysis of histologic follow-up and risk of malignancy for salivary gland neoplasm of uncertain malignant potential proposed by the Milan system for reporting salivary gland cytopathology. Cancer Cytopathol 2018;126(7):490–7.
37. Liu CC, Jethwa AR, Khariwala SS, et al. Sensitivity, specificity, and posttest probability of parotid fine-needle aspiration: a systematic review and meta-analysis. Otolaryngol Head Neck Surg 2016;154(1):9–23.
38. Witt BL, Schmidt RL. Ultrasound-guided core needle biopsy of salivary gland lesions: a systematic review and meta-analysis. Laryngoscope 2014;124(3): 695–700.
39. Barbarite E, Puram SV, Derakhshan A, et al. A call for universal acceptance of the Milan system for reporting salivary gland cytopathology. Laryngoscope 2020; 130(1):80–5.
40. Pusztaszeri M, Baloch Z, Vielh P, et al. Application of the Milan system for reporting risk stratification in salivary gland cytopathology. Cancer Cytopathol 2018; 126(1):69–70.
41. Faquin WC, Rossi ED, Baloch ZE. The Milan system for reporting salivary gland cytopathology. Cham (Switzerland): Springer; 2018.

42. Forner D, Lee DJ, Walsh C, et al. Outpatient versus inpatient parotidectomy: a systematic review and meta-analysis. Otolaryngol Head Neck Surg 2020; 162(6):818–25.

43. Guntinas-Lichius O, Klussmann JP, Wittekindt C, et al. Parotidectomy for benign parotid disease at a university teaching hospital: outcome of 963 operations. Laryngoscope 2006;116(4):534–40.

44. Koch M, Zenk J, Iro H. Long-term results of morbidity after parotid gland surgery in benign disease. Laryngoscope 2010;120(4):724–30.

45. Klintworth N, Zenk J, Koch M, et al. Postoperative complications after extracapsular dissection of benign parotid lesions with particular reference to facial nerve function. Laryngoscope 2010;120(3):484–90.

46. Mantsopoulos K, Koch M, Klintworth N, et al. Evolution and changing trends in surgery for benign parotid tumors. Laryngoscope 2015;125(1):122–7.

47. Upton DC, McNamar JP, Connor NP, et al. Parotidectomy: ten-year review of 237 cases at a single institution. Otolaryngol - Head Neck Surg 2007;136(5):788–92.

48. Neuman MD, Bosk CL. What we talk about when we talk about risk: refining surgery's hazards in medical thought. Milbank Q 2012;90(1):135–59.

49. Sacks GD, Dawes AJ, Ettner SL, et al. Surgeon perception of risk and benefit in the decision to operate. Ann Surg 2016;264(6):896–903.

50. Li G, Warner M, Lang BH, et al. Epidemiology of anesthesia-related mortality in the United States, 1999-2005. Anesthesiology 2009;110(4):759–65.

51. Ferrier MB, Spuesens EB, Le Cessie S, et al. Comorbidity as a major risk factor for mortality and complications in head and neck surgery. Arch Otolaryngol Head Neck Surg 2005;131(1):27–32.

52. Gregory Farwell D, Reilly DF, Weymuller EA, et al. Predictors of perioperative complications in head and neck patients. Arch Otolaryngol Head Neck Surg 2002;128(5):505–11.

53. Bilen-Rosas G, Karanikolas M, Evers A, et al. Impact of anesthesia management characteristics on severe morbidity and mortality: are we convinced? [5]. Anesthesiology 2006;104(1):204.

54. Cheung SH, Kwan WYW, Tsui KP, et al. Partial parotidectomy under local anesthesia for benign parotid tumors: an experience of 50 cases. Am J Otolaryngol 2018;39(3):286–9.

55. Kligerman MP, Jin M, Ayoub N, et al. Comparison of parotidectomy with observation for treatment of pleomorphic adenoma in adults. JAMA Otolaryngol Head Neck Surg 2020;146(11):1027–34.

56. ACS-NSQIP Risk Calculator. American College of Surgeons National Surgical Quality Improvement Program. Available at: http://riskcalculator.facs.org/RiskCalculator/. Accessed May 1, 2021.

57. Bilimoria KY, Liu Y, Paruch JL, et al. Surgical risk calculator: a decision aide and informed consent tool for patients and surgeons. J Am Coll Surg 2013;217(5):833–42.e3.

58. Sacks GD, Dawes AJ, Ettner SL, et al. Impact of a risk calculator on risk perception and surgical decision making: a randomized trial. Ann Surg 2016;264(6):889–95.

59. Marin VTW, Salmaso R, Onnis GL. Tumors of salivary glands. Review of 479 cases with particular reference to histological types, site, age and sex distribution. Appl Pathol 1989;7(3):154–60.

60. Pinkston JA, Cole P. Incidence rates of salivary gland tumors: results from a population-based study. Otolaryngol Head Neck Surg 1999;120(6):834–40.

61. Eneroth CM. Salivary gland tumors in the parotid gland, submandibular gland, and the palate region. Cancer 1971;27(6):1415–8.
62. El-Naggar AK, Chan JKC, Rubin Grandis J, et al, WHO classification of head and neck tumours. International Agency for Research on Cancer (IARC), Lyon, France 2017.
63. Hellquist H, Paiva-Correia A, Vander Poorten V, et al. Analysis of the clinical relevance of histological classification of benign epithelial salivary gland tumours. Adv Ther 2019;36(8):1950–74.
64. Nouraei SAR, Ferguson MS, Clarke PM, et al. Metastasizing pleomorphic salivary adenoma. Arch Otolaryngol Head Neck Surg 2006;132(7):788–93.
65. Marioni G, Marino F, Stramare R, et al. Benign metastasizing pleomorphic adenoma of the parotid gland: a clinicopathologic puzzle. Head Neck 2003;25(12): 1071–6.
66. Antony J, Gopalan V, Smith RA, et al. Carcinoma ex pleomorphic adenoma: a comprehensive review of clinical, pathological and molecular data. Head Neck Pathol 2012;6(1):1–9.
67. Tortoledo ME, Luna MA, Batsakis JG. Carcinomas ex pleomorphic adenoma and malignant mixed tumors. Histomorphologic indexes. Arch Otolaryngol 1984; 110(3):172–6.
68. Olsen KD, Lewis JE. Carcinoma ex pleomorphic adenoma: a clinicopathologic review. Head Neck 2001;23(9):705–12.
69. Witt RL, Eisele DW, Morton RP, et al. Etiology and management of recurrent parotid pleomorphic adenoma. Laryngoscope 2015;125(4):888–93.
70. Kanatas A, Ho MWS, Mücke T. Current thinking about the management of recurrent pleomorphic adenoma of the parotid: a structured review. Br J Oral Maxillofac Surg 2018;56(4):243–8.

Management Options for Sialadenosis

Andrew B. Davis, MD*, Henry T. Hoffman, MD

KEYWORDS

- Sialadenosis • Sialosis • Parotid gland swelling • Bilateral parotid gland swelling

KEY POINTS

- Sialadenosis (sialosis) is a chronic, noninflammatory, nonneoplastic, bilateral, often painless enlargement of the salivary glands, most frequently affecting the parotid glands.
- Approximately 50% of cases are associated with an underlying disease process.
- The pathogenesis of sialadenosis is unknown but likely results from an autonomic neuropathy.
- The key to management is diagnosis and management of any poorly controlled underlying medical process.

INTRODUCTION

Sialadenosis (sialosis) is a rare condition that is defined as noninflammatory, nonneoplastic, bilateral, parenchymatous enlargement of the salivary glands.[1–9] Sialadenosis preferentially affects the parotid glands; however, all other salivary glands may be involved. Sialadenosis is characterized by chronic swelling that is largely painless. Half of all cases of sialadenosis are associated with a recognized endocrine, metabolic, neurogenic, or nutritional disorder.[8] The multiple number of disparate options that have been proposed for management of sialadenosis reflects both the absence of a single effective treatment and also an incomplete understanding of the pathophysiology. A discussion of uncertainties regarding the diagnosis and cause is needed to interpret recommendations regarding the management of sialadenosis.

PATHOPHYSIOLOGY

Sialadenosis is associated with a wide range of disease processes. As a result, identification of a clear pathophysiology has been difficult. A leading hypothesis was proposed by Donath and Seifert.[10] They found the parotid glands of patients with sialosis were characterized by enlargement of acinar cells with an increase in number of secretory granules compared with controls. They also noted degenerative changes of the myoepithelial cells and post–ganglionic sympathetic nerves in the specimens examined. Their conclusions

Otolaryngology Department, University of Iowa Hospitals and Clinics, Iowa City, IA, USA
* Corresponding author.
E-mail address: andrew-davis-2@uiowa.edu

Otolaryngol Clin N Am 54 (2021) 605–611
https://doi.org/10.1016/j.otc.2021.02.005
0030-6665/21/© 2021 Elsevier Inc. All rights reserved.

oto.theclinics.com

were that sialadenosis arises from an autonomic neuropathy associated with dysfunctional protein secretion and/or synthesis, which causes acinar enlargement and buildup of secretory granules.[1,4,10] This hypothesis has been used to explain why metabolic disease processes with known autonomic neuropathies, such as diabetes, have a high rate of sialadenosis.[5,7,11] Association of sialadenosis with other disease processes, such as bulimia, liver disease, alcoholism, and obesity, has led to other proposed mechanisms for the salivary gland enlargement seen with sialadenosis.[12,13]

EVALUATION

Sialadenosis is characterized by a chronic, bilateral swelling of the salivary glands that preferentially affects the parotid glands. It is often persistent and unassociated with signs of inflammation. The differential diagnosis of salivary swelling is broad. There are several other diagnoses that may mimic sialadenosis that require investigation.

The classic sialadenosis patient complains of chronic bilateral parotid swelling (although other glands can be involved) with concern for aesthetic disfigurement. In many instances, the aesthetic disfigurement is the chief complaint for the consultation. Other symptoms, such as xerostomia and pain, may be reported, which, when present, warrant broadening the differential diagnosis to expand the evaluation.[4,11] Metabolic and nutritional diseases have been described as the main players in sialadenosis, with malnutrition, liver disease/cirrhosis (often alcohol related), and diabetes being the most defined causes.

Malnutrition disorders, such as bulimia and anorexia nervosa, were identified as a cause for sialadenosis in 1969.[14] It has been estimated that 10% to 66% of all bulimics have sialadenosis, with unclear pathogenesis.[15] A leading theory that has been proposed is that the glandular hypertrophy occurs because of repetitive autonomic stimulation during purging. Irrespective of its pathogenesis, bulimics who do suffer from sialadenosis are of special concern, because these patients have significant body image issues. Bulimics tend to have glandular swelling a few days after a binge-purge episode. After chronic purging, it can take years for the glandular hypertrophy to resolve, if it ever completely does. There also is an extremely high recurrence rate of sialadenosis in bulimics, because of the high recurrence of bulimia itself.[15]

Alcoholism and alcoholic cirrhosis are well-known causes of sialadenosis, with 30% to 80% of alcoholic cirrhotics and 26% to 86% of alcoholics having sialadenosis.[5,7,16] Autonomic polyneuropathy in alcoholism is well documented. but there is controversy regarding an association between sialadenosis and nonalcoholic liver disease. A study of 28 liver-transplant patients with sialadenosis showed that 17 had non-alcohol-related liver disease. This finding confounds the idea that alcohol itself is the underlying causative agent of sialadenosis. What could potentially be occurring is that the nutritional deficits present in patients with alcoholism and liver disease are the driver of sialadenosis.[16]

It should be noted that because many of the disease processes that cause sialadenosis overlap, there is not always a clear, single, cause. For example, the liver is essential for glucose and glycogen metabolism. As a result, liver disease may result in metabolic derangements, such as hyperglycemia and insulin resistance. These associations make it difficult to establish whether cirrhosis or the subsequent diabetes is the major underlying factor.[16] It has been estimated that 49% of patients with sialadenosis have diabetes. It is also important to note that along with diabetes, the rising epidemic of obesity and subsequent metabolic syndrome is a known cause of sialadenosis. There has been a significant correlation between body mass index and parotid gland size.[17,18]

IMAGING

Ultrasound, computed tomography (CT), and sialography are the most common imaging modalities used to identify sialadenosis. These modalities can be useful in narrowing down the bilateral parotid swelling differential diagnosis. Ultrasound of the salivary glands is a relatively inexpensive and easily obtainable imaging modality helping the initial evaluation to narrow the differential diagnosis. Specifically, in sialadenosis, it is important to confirm that the bilateral swelling is not of inflammatory or neoplastic origins. In cases of sialadenosis, the glandular structure generally shows hyperechogenicity with no focal lesions present.[19]

CT may be more specific in establishing a diagnosis of sialadenosis but does require appropriate clinical correlations. Initially, in sialadenosis, CT will show diffuse glandular enlargement, which will give way to fatty infiltration as the process becomes more chronic (**Fig. 1**).[7,20,21] This glandular enlargement is observed in the absence of identification of other causes, such as stone, tumor, or duct obstruction.

Sialography has had a controversial role in sialadenosis.[22] Sialography is more useful for diagnosis of later stage sialadenosis because of a characteristic appearance of thin ductal system, secondary to parenchymal swelling. The larger the glandular hypertrophy is, the smaller the ductal system is. In extreme cases, there may be no visualization of the proximal (intraglandular) ductal system. This classic sialography finding in sialadenosis has been termed "leafless tree pattern" (**Fig. 2**).[3]

Pathologic analysis is not frequently used for diagnosis of sialadenosis but does have characteristic findings of acinar enlargement and granular appearance to its cytoplasm and can be used to rule out associated tumor (**Fig. 3**).[10] Diagnostic criteria

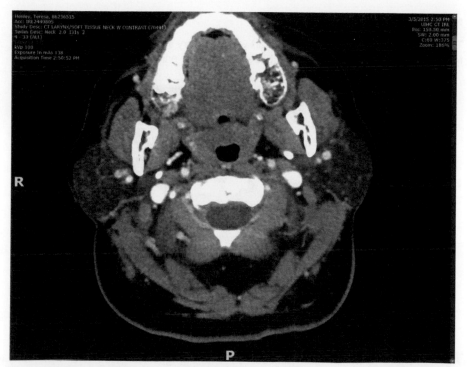

Fig. 1. CT scan of sialadenosis showing characteristic bilateral parotid gland enlargement.

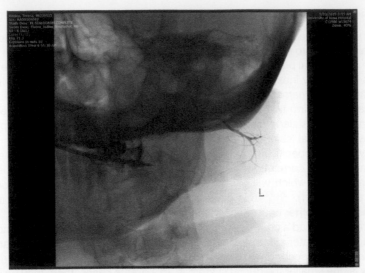

Fig. 2. Sialography on a patient with sialadenosis. This sialogram shows characteristic findings of a "leafless tree pattern" or of a thin, hairline salivary ductal system secondary to external compression.

for acinar enlargement on a fine needle aspiration sample have been proposed at 62 μM.[21] Studies have also shown the pathologic findings of myoepithelial cell degeneration in sialadenosis.[4]

MANAGEMENT

The work up of sialadenosis should start with a history and physical examination looking for any underlying cause of bilateral parotid enlargement.[22–24] On physical

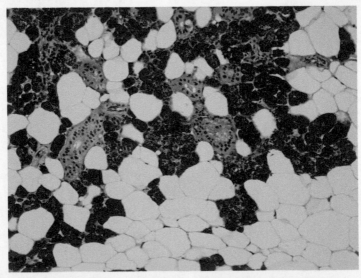

Fig. 3. Parotid specimen with sialadenosis showing glandular structure with fatty infiltration.

examination, the parotid enlargement commonly results in obliteration of the groove between the ramus of the mandible and mastoid process causing a trapezoid appearance.[17] A combination of laboratory tests, imaging, and pathologic assessment may be needed for proper identification of underlying cause and also to rule out other causes of bilateral parotid enlargement. Regardless of confirmation of the underlying disease process, resolution of the swelling is variable.[3,15] Initial management options need to concentrate on resolving the underlying disease processes.

Metabolic and nutritional disorders are the culprits in most sialadenosis patients. Patients with bulimia and anorexia have a particularly difficult time with resolution of sialadenosis because of the difficulty of curing the underlying eating disorder. Treatment starts with psychiatric therapy in an attempt to control the purging behaviors. It is reported that only 50% of patients with bulimia are recovered at 10 years. Because of the difficulty in curing the disease process, the salivary swelling in these patients tends to be chronic, requiring months of no purging behaviors.[25]

Alcoholism with liver disease is classically associated with sialadenosis, likely because of the fact that these patients have severe liver damage causing significant nutritional and metabolic deficits. All patients with disease processes that can cause malnutrition can lead to sialadenosis. First-line treatment in these cases is cessation of the hepatotoxic agent and correction of the nutritional and metabolic deficiencies.

Beyond treatment of the underlying cause, conservative options are present, with the goal of decreasing the patient's symptom burden. Patients can perform heat application, massage, and sialogogues to stimulate salivary flow in an attempt to decrease salivary swelling. Salivary substitutes can also be used in patients who have sialadenosis and xerostomia. Pilocarpine, which is a nonselective muscarinic agonist with a mild B-adrenergic, has been shown to increase salivary flow in patients with sialadenosis and xerostomia, and in some cases, resolved the swelling that was present.[26,27] It has also been reported to potentially decrease the salivary swelling in patients with bulimia.[15] Reports are mixed on the benefits of salivary stimulants in sialadenosis. The use of pilocarpine should only be started after an assessment of the patient's comorbidities owing to its side-effect profile, which includes sweating, nausea, rhinorrhea, flushing, and dizziness.

Surgical management is usually held as a last resort for refractory cases when the aesthetic appearance of the glandular swelling is unacceptable. Because of comorbidities associated with sialadenosis, assessment of the patient's ability to undergo surgical treatment should be performed, and consultation with medical and psychiatric specialties should be used.[25] Some investigators do not recommend surgical management in specific patient groups, such as bulimics, because of their severe body image issues and the potential of morbidity and poor aesthetic results with the surgery.[15,25] If surgical treatment is performed in bulimics, long-term follow-up must be maintained, because of the high recurrence rate of sialadenosis in these patients.[25]

Tympanic neurectomy is a surgical treatment that involves denervating the parotid gland of parasympathetic innervation, which causes subsequent glandular atrophy. Patients initially have decreased glandular swelling, but in some cases, swelling recurs, likely secondary to parasympathetic reinnervation.[21] Botulinum neurotoxin injection has been used in cases to cause atrophy to the offending gland; however, this procedure must be repeated to obtain consistent results. Parotidectomy, although curative, is deemed as a last resort because of the more extensive surgery and potential for complications. After surgical resection, the lack of volume in the cheek region can lead to other aesthetic concerns, especially in patients with body image issues, although this can be addressed at the time of surgery using various reconstructive options. Also, an extensive informed consent process must occur, because of potential damage to the facial nerve. Some groups do advocate for superficial parotidectomy in specific situations having shown adequate cosmetic results.[25]

CLINICS CARE POINTS

- Sialadenosis requires an initial clinical evaluation consisting of a thorough history and physical examination to direct further investigation that may include blood testing to narrow the large differential diagnosis characterizing bilateral parotid swelling.

- Diagnostic imaging, including ultrasound, computed tomography, and sialography, is useful in supporting the diagnosis of sialadenosis.

- Fine needle aspiration biopsy may be required to exclude tumor and may provide evidence of large ($\geq$62 μm) acini consistent with sialadenosis.

- Initial management involves treating the underlying clinical condition causing sialadenosis. Complete resolution of the glandular swelling is variable.

- Conservative measures, including observation, should be considered as initial management. More invasive management is reserved for refractory cases.

DISCLOSURE

H.T. Hoffman: COOK Medical Research Consultant, *UpToDate* author. A.B. Davis: None.

REFERENCES

1. Ascoli V, Albedi FM, De Blasiis R, et al. Sialadenosis of the parotid gland: report of four cases diagnosed by fine-needle aspiration cytology. Diagn Cytopathol 1993; 9(2):151–5.
2. Batsakis JG. Pathology consultation. Sialadenosis. Ann Otol Rhinol Laryngol 1988;97(1):94–5.
3. Coleman H, Altini M, Nayler S, et al. Sialadenosis: a presenting sign in bulimia. Head Neck 1998;20(8):758–62.
4. Ihrler S, Rath C, Zengel P, et al. Pathogenesis of sialadenosis: possible role of functionally deficient myoepithelial cells. Oral Surg Oral Med Oral Pathol Oral Radiol Endod 2010;110(2):218–23.
5. Kastin B, Mandel L. Alcoholic sialosis. N Y State Dent J 2000;66(6):22–4.
6. Kim D, Uy C, Mandel L. Sialosis of unknown origin. N Y State Dent J 1998;64(7): 38–40.
7. Mandel L, Baurmash H. Parotid enlargement due to alcoholism. J Am Dent Assoc 1971;82(2):369–73.
8. Butt F. Benign diseases of the salivary glands. Chapter 18. In: Lalwani AK, editor. CURRENT diagnosis & treatment in Otolaryngology—Head & Neck surgery. 3rd edition. New York: McGraw-Hill; 2012. Available at: http://accessmedicine.mhmedical.com. proxy.lib.uiowa.edu/content.aspx?bookid=386&Sectionid=39944053. Accessed February 24, 2016.
9. Dhillon N. Anatomy. Chapter 1. In: Lalwani AK, editor. Current diagnosis & treatment in otolaryngology—head & neck surgery. 3rd edition. New York: McGraw-Hill; 2012. Available at: http://accessmedicine.mhmedical.com.proxy.lib.uiowa. edu/content.aspx?bookid=386&Sectionid=39944032. Accessed February 24, 2016.

10. Donath K, Seifert G. Ultrastructural studies of the parotid glands in sialadenosis. Virchows Arch A Pathol Anat Histol 1975;365(2):119–35.
11. Merlo C, Bohl L, Carda C, et al. Parotid sialosis: morphometrical analysis of the glandular parenchyme and stroma among diabetic and alcoholic patients. J Oral Pathol Med 2010;39(1):10–5.
12. Mandic R, Teymoortash A, Kann PH, et al. Sialadenosis of the major salivary glands in a patient with central diabetes insipidus–implications of aquaporin water channels in the pathomechanism of sialadenosis. Exp Clin Endocrinol Diabetes 2005;113(4):205–7.
13. Teymoortash A, Wiegand S, Borkeloh M, et al. Variations in the expression and distribution pattern of AQP5 in acinar cells of patients with sialadenosis. In Vivo 2012;26:951–6.
14. Lavender S. Vomiting and parotid enlargement. Lancet 1969;1:426.
15. Mehler PS, Wallace JA. Sialadenosis in bulimia. A new treatment. Arch Otolaryngol Head Neck Surg 1993;119(7):787–8.
16. Guggenheimer J, Close JM, Eghtesad B. Sialadenosis in patients with advanced liver disease. Head Neck Pathol 2009;3(2):100–5.
17. Scully C, Bagán JV, Eveson JW, et al. Sialosis: 35 cases of persistent parotid swelling from two countries. Br J Oral Maxillofac Surg 2008;46(6):468–72.
18. Bozzato A, Burger P, Zenk J, et al. Salivary gland biometry in female patients with eating disorders. Eur Arch Otorhinolaryngol 2008;265(9):1095–102.
19. Gritzmann N, Rettenbacher T, Hollerweger A, et al. Sonography of the salivary glands. Eur Radiol 2003;13(5):964–75.
20. Whyte AM, Bowyer FM. Sialosis: diagnosis by computed tomography. Br J Radiol 1987;60(712):400–1.
21. Pape SA, MacLeod RI, McLean NR, et al. Sialadenosis of the salivary glands. Br J Plast Surg 1995;48(6):419–22.
22. Morgan RF, Saunders JR Jr, Hirata RM, et al. A comparative analysis of the clinical, sialographic, and pathologic findings in parotid disease. Am Surg 1985; 51(11):664–7.
23. Borsanyi SJ, Blanchard CL. Asymptomatic parotid swelling and isoproterenol. Laryngoscope 1962;72:1777–83.
24. Mauz PS, Mörike K, Kaiserling E, et al. Valproic acid-associated sialadenosis of the parotid and submandibular glands: diagnostic and therapeutic aspects. Acta Otolaryngol 2005;125(4):386–91.
25. Garcia Garcia B, Dean Ferrer A, Diaz Jimenez N, et al. Bilateral parotid sialadenosis associated with long-standing bulimia: a case report and literature review. J Maxillofac Oral Surg 2018;17(2):117–21.
26. Aframian DJ, Helcer M, Livni D, et al. Pilocarpine treatment in a mixed cohort of xerostomic patients. Oral Dis 2007;13(1):88–92.
27. Hoffman, H (ed) Iowa Head and Neck Protocols. Sialosis or sialadenosis case example of surgical treatment. Available at: https://iowaheadneckprotocols.oto. uiowa.edu/display/protocols/Sialosis+or+sialadenosis+Case+example+of+ surgical+treatment. Accessed February 29, 2016.

SALIVARY MALIGNANCY

Molecular Markers that Matter in Salivary Malignancy

Katherine C. Wai, MD[a], Hyunseok Kang, MD[b], Patrick K. Ha, MD[a],*

KEYWORDS

- Salivary gland cancer • Targeted therapy • Molecular markers

KEY POINTS

- Salivary gland cancers remain a challenging, heterogeneous group of tumors to treat, despite advances in targeted therapy.
- Many molecular markers have been tested, including several in the tyrosine kinase receptor family, androgen receptor, Notch signaling pathway, epigenetics via histone deacetylase, and immunotherapy (programmed cell death protein 1), all of which have shown varying degrees of clinical benefit in phase II clinical trials.
- A majority of targeted therapeutics result in, at least, stabilization of disease in patients with unresectable locally advanced or metastatic salivary gland malignancies, who often have progressed on prior treatments.
- There are several ongoing clinical trials involving previously tested molecular targets as well as novel therapeutics not yet utilized in salivary gland cancers.

INTRODUCTION

Salivary gland cancers (SGCs) represent approximately 5% of head and neck cancers. Despite their rarity, there are a multitude of histologic subtypes.[1] Given the high degree of heterogeneity, standardization of treatment is challenging. Surgery followed by adjuvant radiation for adverse pathologic features is the mainstay of treatment.[2] Unfortunately, locoregional recurrence and metastatic disease are common, despite aggressive initial interventions.[3] Standard chemotherapies have modest responses at best.[4]

There has been a focus toward defining molecular aberrations in SGCs in hopes of generating targeted therapies.[5–7] Several potential biologic targets have been reported. The rationale often is based on specific molecular markers in a particular histologic subtype. Given the rarity of SGCs, however, many early-phase clinical trials include all types

[a] Department of Otolaryngology–Head and Neck Surgery, University of California San Francisco 550 16th Street, 6th floor, UCSF Box 3213, San Francisco, CA 94158, USA; [b] Department of Hematology and Oncology, University of California San Francisco, 1825 4th Street, San Francisco, CA 94158, USA
* Corresponding author.
E-mail address: Patrick.Ha@ucsf.edu

Otolaryngol Clin N Am 54 (2021) 613–627
https://doi.org/10.1016/j.otc.2021.01.007
0030-6665/21/© 2021 Elsevier Inc. All rights reserved.

of SGCs in patients with locally advanced, recurrent, or metastatic disease. The aim of this review is to discuss molecular markers that have been tested as targeted therapeutics in SGCs. The trials discussed in this review are summarized in **Table 1**, with tumor response defined RECIST (response evaluation criteria in solid tumors), version 1.1, guidelines.[8] When evaluating the data, it is important to note that stable disease (SD) may not be a good indicator of response in SGCs, because some of them may have inherently indolent disease courses (in particular, adenoid cystic carcinoma [ACC]).

DISCUSSION
Tyrosine Kinase Pathway

The receptor tyrosine kinase (RTK) family includes a broad range of receptors for cell regulation and survival, with the signaling pathway depicted in **Fig. 1**. Many studies target different receptors within this family.

c-kit receptor

The c-kit receptor is a transmembrane RTK. Upon activation, c-kit has many downstream regulatory effects, including cell proliferation, differentiation, and survival.[9] Approximately 80% of ACCs overexpress c-kit.[10] Imatinib, a small molecule inhibitor of c-kit and platelet-derived growth factor receptor (PDGFR), was tested in multiple clinical trials among patients with recurrent/metastatic (R/M) ACC with little benefit.[11–13] More recently, a phase II trial with dasatinib, a multikinase inhibitor with activity against c-kit, vascular endothelial growth factor receptor (VEGFR), and fibroblast growth factor receptor (FGFR), was tested in patients with c-kit–positive ACC, with only 1 partial response (PR), suggesting c-kit may not be a valid target for ACC.[14]

Epidermal growth factor receptor

Epidermal growth factor receptor (EGFR) activation leads to cell survival and proliferation. Preclinical studies have shown up to 90% of ACCs exhibit high expression of EGFR. Cetuximab, an IgG monoclonal antibody against EGFR, has been used in head and neck squamous cell carcinoma (HNSCC) in combination with radiation and chemotherapy with some success.[15] The only phase II clinical trial with cetuximab for R/M SGCs, however, demonstrated no objective responses.[16] There was no correlation between EGFR expression and clinical response in this study, which is consistent with what is seen in HNSCC. Gefitinib, a small molecule inhibitor of EGFR, was tested in patients with R/M ACC and non-ACC. No objective responses were recorded. Furthermore, progression-free survival (PFS) and overall survival (OS) did not correlate with EGFR or human EGFR 2 (HER2) overexpression.[17] Similar results were observed in a separate clinical trial with gefitinib (NCT00509002) and lapatinib, a dual inhibitor of EGFR and HER2.[18]

Human epidermal growth factor receptor

SGCs overexpress HER2 with varying degrees of prevalence.[19] Trastuzumab and pertuzumab are monoclonal antibodies with different binding sites against HER2. An early trial showed that in patients with R/M SGC with HER2-positive overexpression, only 1/13 patients treated with trastuzumab had a PR.[20] Case series and reports have suggested, however, that HER2-directed therapy in combination with chemotherapy may lead to improved results.[21,22] A larger retrospective study showed that patients with greater expression of HER2-positive SGCs had improved OS and disease-free survival when treated with chemotherapy and adjuvant trastuzumab compared with chemotherapy alone.[23] A phase II clinical trial of patients with unresectable, R/M HER2-positive salivary duct carcinoma (SDC) were treated with both trastuzumab and docetaxel.[24] Of 57 patients, 32 (56%) had PR and 8 (15%) had complete response (CR).

Table 1
Summary of molecular targets in clinical trials

Reference	Drug	Molecular Marker	Patient Population	Phase	Complete Response	Partial Response	Stable Disease	Progression of Disease	Median Overall Survival (Months)	Median Progression-free Survival (Months)
Tyrosine kinase pathway										
Hotte et al,[11] 2005	Imatinib	c-kit, PDGFR	Unresectable or metastatic c-kit + ACC	II	0%	0%	Not reported	Not reported	7.5	2.5
Pfeffer et al,[12] 2007	Imatinib	c-kit, PDGFR	Unresectable or metastatic ACC	II	0%	0%	7%	93%	Not reported	Not reported
Ghosal et al,[13] 2011	Imatinib + cisplatin	c-kit, PDGFR	Unresectable or metastatic c-kit + ACC	II	0%	0%	74%	21%	35	15
Wong et al,[14] 2016	Dasatinib	c-kit	Unresectable ACC with evidence of disease progression in last 4 mo, must be c-kit positive	II	0%	2.50%	50%	48%	14.5	4.8
Locati et al,[16] 2009	Cetuximab	EGFR	R/M SGC	II	0%	0%	80%	20%	Not reported	6.0
Jakob et al,[17] 2015	Gefitinib	EGFR	R/M SGC	II	0%	0%	Not reported	Not reported	ACC (25.9), non-ACC (16)	ACC (4.4), non-ACC (2.1)
Takahashi et al,[24] 2019	Trastuzumab + taxol	HER2	Unresectable R/M SDC	II	14%	56%	25%	2%	39.7	8.9

(continued on next page)

Table 1
(*continued*)

Reference	Drug	Molecular Marker	Patient Population	Phase	Complete Response	Partial Response	Stable Disease	Progression of Disease	Median Overall Survival (Months)	Median Progression-free Survival (Months)
Kurzrock et al,[25] 2020	Trastuzumab, pertuzumab	HER2	All HER2+ SGC	II	7%	53%	7%	33%	20.4	8.6
Ho et al,[31] 2016	Axitinib	VEGFR	Incurable ACC with evidence of disease progression	II	0%	9%	75%	16%	21.8	5.7
Locati et al,[32] 2019	Axitinib	VEGFR	R/M SGC	II	0%	8%	50%	42%	26.2	5.5
Kim et al,[34] 2017	Nintedanib	VEGFR, PDGFR, FGFR	R/M SGC with evidence of disease progression at time of enrollment	II	0%	0%	75%	20%	>12	>6
Keam et al,[39] 2015	Dovitinib	FGFR	Unresectable or metastatic ACC	II	0%	3%	94%	3%	>14	6.0
Dillon et al,[40] 2017	Dovitinib	FGFR	Unresectable or metastatic ACC with evidence of progression in last 6 mo	II	0%	6%	65%	29%	20.6	8.2
Thomson et al,[42] 2015	Sorafenib	Multiple	Unresectable, R/M ACC	II	0%	11%	68%	21%	19.6	11.3
Locati et al,[43] 2016	Sorafenib	Multiple	R/M SGC	II	0%	16%	59%	25%	23.4	5.9

Study	Drug	Target	Patient population	Phase						
Chau et al,[44] 2012	Sunitinib	Multiple	R/M ACC with evidence of progression within 6 mo of enrollment	II	0%	0%	78%	22%	18.7	7.2
Tchekmedyian et al,[46] 2019	Lenvatinib	Multiple	R/M ACC with evidence of progression within 6 mo of enrollment	II	0%	16%	75%	6%	Not reported	17.5
Androgen axis pathway										
Fushimi et al,[60] 2018	Leuprorelin + bicalutamide	AR	Unresectable or R/M AR + SGC	II	11%	31%	44%	14%	30.5	8.8
Notch signaling pathway										
Even et al,[66] 2020	Crenigacestat	Notch	Locally advanced/ metastatic ACC	I	0%	0%	68%	23%	Not reported	5.3
Programmed cell death protein 1 pathway										
Cohen et al,[71] 2018	Pembrolizumab	PD-1	Unresectable or metastatic SGC (any subtype)	I	0%	12%	46%	42%	13.0	4.0
Fayette et al,[73] 2019	Nivolumab	PD-1	Unresectable or metastatic SGC (any subtype)	II	0%	6%	51%	NA	Not reported	Not reported
Rodriguez et al,[77] 2020	Pembrolizumab + vorinostat	PD-1, histone deacetylase	SGC with progression	II	0%	16%	56%	28%	14	6.9
Histone deacetylase										
Goncalves et al,[78] 2020	Vorinostat	Histone deacetylase	Unresectable R/M ACC	II	0%	6%	90%	4%	11.5	10

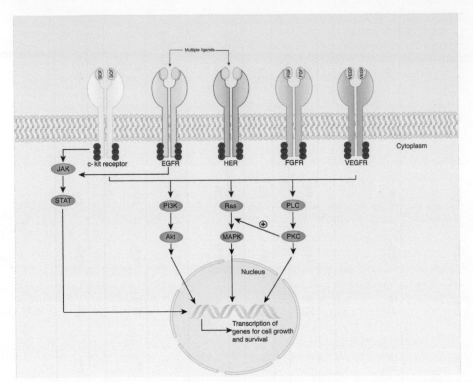

Fig. 1. Tyrosine kinase pathway. RTKs are activated via dimerization of the transmembrane receptors in the presence of different ligands. This interaction results in kinase activation and autophosphorylation, which leads to downstream activation of several signal transduction pathways, ultimately resulting in transcription of genes for cell growth and survival.

An ongoing trial (NCT02091141) reported findings in a subgroup of patients with HER2-positive SGC who were treated with combination blockade, both pertuzumab and trastuzumab.[25] Combination blockade has been shown to be synergistic in HER2-positive breast cancer because pertuzumab binds a different epitope than trastuzumab and prevents the heterodimerization of HER2.[26] Of 15 patients with advanced HER2-positive SGC, 1 had CR, 8 PR, and 1 SD, with median duration response of 9.2 months. A separate phase II trial studied the efficacy of ado-trastuzumab emtansine, an antibody-conjugate therapeutic; emtansine is a cytotoxic agent that prevents microtubule formation. There was an overall response rate (ORR) of 90% in 10 patients with HER2-positive SDC.[27]

Vascular endothelial growth factor receptor

The VEGFR family has an important role in angiogenesis and lymphangiogenesis in cancer; thus, it remains an area of active research for targeted anticancer therapy.[28] High expression of VEGFR in ACC has been associated with worse survival.[29]

Based on in vitro studies, axitinib is thought to be primarily an inhibitor of VEGFR, thereby inhibiting signal transduction of VEGFR and downstream angiogenesis.[30] One phase II trial, which included patients with incurable ACC, found that on axitinib, 9% had a PR and 75% had SD for greater than 6 months.[31] In a separate study using axitinib for ACC and non-ACC subtypes, the investigators found 2/26 (8%) had PR and 13/26 (50%) had SD.[32] In both studies, however, the primary endpoint was not met; thus, the data must be interpreted with caution. One randomized phase II trial of patients with R/M ACC demonstrated that those who received axitinib had improved 6-month PFS compared with observation (10.8 vs 2.8 months, respectively; P<.001), although there was no objective response in axitinib arm.[33]

In addition to VEGFR, PDGFR and FGFR are important for the proangiogenic signaling pathway. Among patients with R/M SGCs who previously failed chemotherapy, nintedanib, a triple-receptor kinase inhibitor of VEGFR, PDGFR, and FGFR, resulted in no objective responses, although 75% exhibited SD.[34]

For patients with R/M ACC, a selective small molecule inhibitor of VEGFR-2, rivoceranib, demonstrated ORR of 47.1% in a phase II study conducted in China.[35] An actively recruiting trial (NCT04119453) using rivoceranib is under way for patients with R/M ACC in the United States.

Fibroblast growth factor receptor

ACCs often acquire a chromosomal translocation that results in the overexpression of MYB,[36] an oncogenic transcription factor. In vitro studies in melanoma found that overexpression of c-MYB mRNA indirectly activates the FGF (fibroblast growth factor)-2 promoter and leads to unregulated cell proliferation.[37] This suggests a possible mechanism for tumorigenesis in ACC and a rationale for investigation as a targeted treatment.

Dovitinib, a multikinase inhibitor, has been tested in phase II clinical trials as an FGFR inhibitor, because studies have shown greater activity against FGFR compared with other small molecule inhibitors.[38] Keam and colleagues delivered dovitinib to locally advanced/metastatic ACCs with the primary endpoint at 4-months PFS. Of 32 patients, 94% had SD and 3% had a PR at greater than 4 months.[39] A more recent study administering dovitinib to unresectable/metastatic ACCs showed similar numbers, with 65% with SD and 6% with PR; but the majority of patients required dose reduction due to side effects.[40]

Another study utilizing regorafenib, a multikinase inhibitor with activity against VEGFR and c-kit, currently is under way for patients with R/M ACC (NCT02098538).

Multiple kinase inhibitor

There also have been several studies involving multikinase inhibitors that have potent activity against a broad range of RTKs rather than more selective inhibition.

Sorafenib targets the Raf serine/threonine kinases and RTKs (VEGFR, PDGFR, Flt-3, and c-kit).[41] When given to 19 patients with R/M ACC in a phase II clinical trial, 2 (11%) had PR and 13 (68%) had SD for at least 6 months.[42] In a broader study, including R/M ACC and non-ACC patients, 16% had PR and 59% experienced SD.[43] This study also included immunohistochemistry (IHC) and molecular analysis from the primary tumor. Among the 6 patients who experienced PR, all had a PDGFR-β–rich stromal component on IHC, suggesting this is the primary mechanism of action of sorafenib in SGC. In contrast, sunitinib, another inhibitor with activity against VEGFR, PDGFR, Flt-3, c-kit, and RET, showed no objective responses.[44]

Lenvatinib is another multikinase inhibitor with activity against VEGFR, FGFR, PDGFR, c-kit, and RET.[45] One phase II trial found showed among 32 patients with R/M ACC with evidence of disease progression at enrollment, 5/32 (16%) showed PR and 24/32 (75%) had SD.[46] MYB IHC was performed on 30/32 tumor specimens. Although not the primary outcome, there was no clear association between MYB overexpression and response rate, which suggests the mechanism of action of VEGFR, PDGFR, Flt-3, c-kit, and RET is independent of this pathway.

Entrectinib and larotrectinib are 2 different small molecule tyrosine kinase inhibitors that specifically target the downstream effects of the abnormal ETV6-NTRK gene rearrangement, often found in secretory carcinomas.[47,48] Although no clinical trials have specifically tested these drugs in secretory carcinoma alone, single-arm studies have shown remarkable clinical benefit in malignancies with confirmed NTRK fusions.[49,50]

Androgen–Androgen Receptor Axis

Androgen receptor (AR) is important in tumorigenesis through its direct DNA binding and subsequent transcription of proteins leading to cell growth and survival (**Fig. 2**).[51] Specifically, 67% to 89% of SDCs overexpress AR.[52,53] Studies have suggested androgen deprivation therapy (ADT), which inhibits the androgen-AR axis, may lead to tumor control.[54–56] A retrospective cohort study in locally advanced or metastatic AR-positive SDCs demonstrated that compared with supportive care, those who received ADT (either bicalutamide or combination goserelin and bicalutamide) had improved OS with a clinical benefit rate of 50% with either SD or PR.[57] Even in the presence of HER2-positivity, patients with AR-positive SDC showed clinical benefit with ADT.[58] Another study that compared ADT with platinum-based chemotherapy regimens found similar OS but improved response rates in the ADT group.[59]

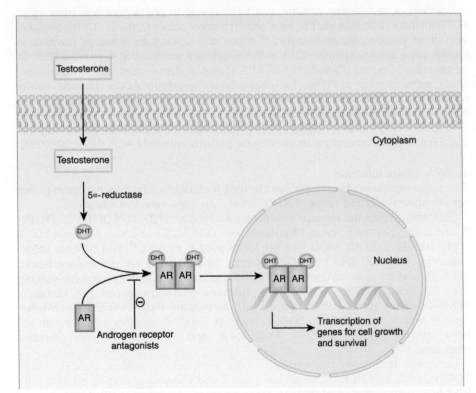

Fig. 2. Androgen axis pathway. Testosterone is converted to dihydrotestosterone (DHT) intracellularly by 5α-reductase. DHT binds to its ligand-binding domain of the AR. AR then dimerizes and translocates to the nucleus, where it binds to its promoter region and activates transcription of genes for cell growth and survival. AR blockers are competitive antagonists of the DHT ligand-binding domain.

In a phase II clinical trial of recurrent or unresectable AR-positive SGC, patients who were treated with ADT, including leuprorelin (luteinizing hormone–releasing hormone agonist) and bicalutamide (AR antagonist) had no objective responses but 75% had SD.[60] Histologic subtypes included SDC (94%) and adenocarcinoma not otherwise specified (6%). One phase II study of monotherapy with enzalutamide, an AR antagonist, did not meet their primary endpoint, with 2/46 PRs after 8 cycles.[61]

A retrospective study suggested benefits of adjuvant ADT in surgically treated poor-risk patients, with 3-year disease-free survival of 48.2% in ADT group versus 27.7% in non-ADT group.[62] Ongoing clinical trials are under way to compare ADT to chemotherapy (NCT01969578) and to determine if there is a synergistic effect between ADT and immune checkpoint inhibition (NCT03942653).

Notch Signaling Pathway

The Notch signaling pathway regulates multiple cellular processes, including proliferation, differentiation, and apoptosis (**Fig. 3**). Notch proteins are transmembrane receptors that activate via ligand binding. Upon activation, the Notch receptor undergoes

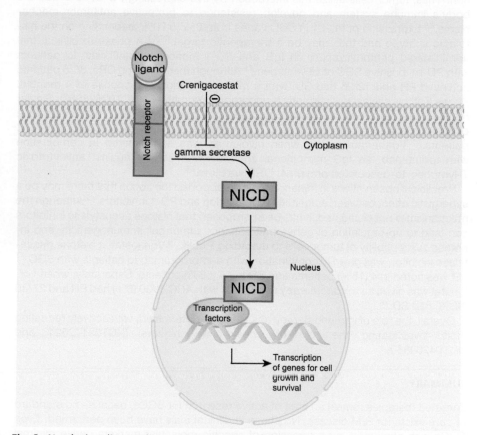

Fig. 3. Notch signaling pathway. Upon binding of the notch ligand to the Notch receptor, the intracellular site undergoes proteolytic cleavage by gamma secretase, resulting in release of the NICD. The NICD translocates to the nucleus and interacts with other transcription factors to activate the production of genes required for cell growth. Crenigacestat is a small molecule inhibitor of gamma secretase that prevents the release of NICD.

cleavage by the gamma secretase complex releasing the Notch intracellular domain (NICD). NICD translocates to the nucleus and drives expression of genes that regulate cell growth and differentiation. Prior work has shown that up-regulation of Notch-1 in patients with ACCs may portend a worse prognosis.[63,64] Furthermore, in vivo Notch-1 knockdown mice models suppressed metastases.[65]

Recently, a phase I clinical trial utilizing Crenigacestat, a small molecule inhibitor of gamma secretase, was tested among patients with advanced/metastatic ACC, with 68% of patients achieving SD but none with objective responses.[66] Currently, there is an ongoing phase II clinical trial using study drug AL101, another small molecule inhibitor of gamma secretase, in patients with ACC with known activating notch mutations. Preliminary data suggest 6/40 PR and 21/40 SD.[67]

Programmed Cell Death Protein 1

Programmed cell death protein 1 (PD-1) is a cell surface receptor commonly expressed on T cells. PD-1, when bound to its ligands, PD-L1 and PD-L2, is tissue protective, blocking the T-cell response, such as cytotoxic ability and cytokine secretion. Thus, tumor cells utilize this interaction by overexpressing PD-L1 to evade the body's immune system and develop resistance to protective antitumor mechanisms.[68] Expression of PD-L1 in SGC varies from 0% to 70%, depending on the histologic subtype and thus may be a therapeutic target.[69,70] A phase Ib clinical trial administered pembrolizumab, an IgG anti–PD-1 monoclonal antibody, to patients with PD-L1-positive SGC of all subtypes.[71] Although there were no CRs, 3/26 patients achieved PR and 12/26 had SD, with a median duration of response of 4 months. Phase II of this clinical trial currently is undergoing recruitment (NCT02628067). Similar results were seen with nivolumab, another IgG inhibitor of PD-1 that binds to a different epitope than pembrolizumab,[72] even when stratified by ACC and non-ACC patients.[73] Furthermore, even when nivolumab was administered in combination with ipilimumab, an IgG monoclonal antibody with activity against anticytotoxic T-lymphocyte–associated protein 4, ORR was low.[74]

Preclinical observations in melanoma have supported the notion that there may be a synergistic effect between epigenetic modification and PD-1 inhibitors.[75] Although the mechanism is not elucidated, it has been proposed that histone deacetylase inhibitors can lead to up-regulation of genes that enhance tumor cell immunogenicity and increase susceptibility of tumor cells to cytotoxic T cells.[76] Vorinostat, a histone deacetylase inhibitor, was given in combination with pembrolizumab to patients with SGC.[77] PR was noted in 4 (16%) patients and SD in 14 (56%) patients. Separately, when vorinostat was given as a monotherapy to patients with ACC, 2/30 (6%) had PR and 27/30 (90%) had SD.[78]

Overall, the role of immunotherapy has yet to be determined, with actively recruiting trials investigating the role of checkpoint inhibitors (NCT03172624 and NCT04209660).

SUMMARY

Targeted therapies remain an area of active research for SGCs, because no standard of care exists for R/M disease. No phase III clinical trials have been performed. Even SGCs with confirmed overexpression of specific molecular markers derive minimal benefit from targeted therapeutics, with the majority resulting in SD at best, and few exceptions inducing objective responses, including drugs targeting AR, HER2, and VEGFR. Beyond the current literature, there are ongoing clinical trials to (1) continue testing the previously described molecular markers, (2) test new molecular targets that reactivate tumor suppression pathways and enhance antitumor activity (NCT03781986, NCT02069730), and (3) evaluate a vaccine carrying the inactivated MYB gene in hopes of helping the immune system recognize malignant cells in MYB overexpressing ACC by evaluating the T-cell immunologic response and clinical benefit response (NCT03287427). Future studies are needed to better understand the molecular portfolio of this heterogeneous group of tumors, in order to improve the success of targeted therapies.

CLINICS CARE POINTS

- Upfront surgery followed by adjuvant radiation remains the primary treatment approach, but, despite aggressive treatment, recurrent and/or metastatic disease remains common in high grade cancers.
- Several salivary gland subtypes express specific molecular markers, and these have been the target of many phase I/II clinical trials.

DISCLOSURES

No relevant commercial or financial conflicts of interest to disclose. No funding sources.

REFERENCES

1. Seethala RR, Stenman G. Update from the 4th edition of the world health organization classification of head and neck tumours: tumors of the salivary gland. Head Neck Pathol 2017;11(1):55–67.
2. National comprehensive cancer network. Salivary gland tumors (Version 2.2020). Available at: https://jnccn.org/view/journals/jnccn/18/7/article-p873.xml. Accessed September 6, 2020.
3. Szewczyk M, Golusiński P, Pazdrowski J, et al. Patterns of treatment failure in salivary gland cancers. Rep Pract Oncol Radiother 2018;23(4):260–5.
4. Lagha A, Chraiet N, Ayadi M, et al. Systemic therapy in the management of metastatic or advanced salivary gland cancers. Head Neck Oncol 2012;4:19.
5. Keller G, Steinmann D, Quaas A, et al. New concepts of personalized therapy in salivary gland carcinomas. Oral Oncol 2017;68:103–13.
6. Schvartsman G, Pinto NA, Bell D, et al. Salivary gland tumors: molecular characterization and therapeutic advances for metastatic disease. Head Neck 2019; 41(1):239–47.
7. Cavalieri S, Platini F, Bergamini C, et al. Genomics in non-adenoid cystic group of salivary gland cancers: one or more druggable entities? Expert Opin Investig Drugs 2019;28(5):435–43.
8. Eisenhauer EA, Therasse P, Bogaerts J, et al. New response evaluation criteria in solid tumours: revised RECIST guideline (version 1.1). Eur J Cancer 2009;45(2): 228–47.
9. Liang J, Wu YL, Chen BJ, et al. The C-kit receptor-mediated signal transduction and tumor-related diseases. Int J Biol Sci 2013;9(5):435–43.
10. Jeng YM, Lin CY, Hsu HC. Expression of the c-kit protein is associated with certain subtypes of salivary gland carcinoma. Cancer Lett 2000;154(1):107–11.
11. Hotte SJ, Winquist EW, Lamont E, et al. Imatinib mesylate in patients with adenoid cystic cancers of the salivary glands expressing c-kit: a princess margaret hospital phase II consortium study. J Clin Oncol 2005;23(3):585–90.

12. Pfeffer MR, Talmi Y, Catane R, et al. A phase II study of Imatinib for advanced adenoid cystic carcinoma of head and neck salivary glands. Oral Oncol 2007; 43(1):33–6.

13. Ghosal N, Mais K, Shenjere P, et al. Phase II study of cisplatin and imatinib in advanced salivary adenoid cystic carcinoma. Br J Oral Maxillofac Surg 2011; 49(7):510–5.

14. Wong SJ, Karrison T, Hayes DN, et al. Phase II trial of dasatinib for recurrent or metastatic c-KIT expressing adenoid cystic carcinoma and for nonadenoid cystic malignant salivary tumors. Ann Oncol 2016;27(2):318–23.

15. Bonner JA, Harari PM, Giralt J, et al. Radiotherapy plus cetuximab for squamous-cell carcinoma of the head and neck. N Engl J Med 2006;354(6):567–78.

16. Locati LD, Bossi P, Perrone F, et al. Cetuximab in recurrent and/or metastatic salivary gland carcinomas: a phase II study. Oral Oncol 2009;45(7):574–8.

17. Jakob JA, Kies MS, Glisson BS, et al. Phase II study of gefitinib in patients with advanced salivary gland cancers. Head Neck 2015;37(5):644–9.

18. Agulnik M, Cohen EW, Cohen RB, et al. Phase II study of lapatinib in recurrent or metastatic epidermal growth factor receptor and/or erbB2 expressing adenoid cystic carcinoma and non adenoid cystic carcinoma malignant tumors of the salivary glands. J Clin Oncol 2007;25(25):3978–84.

19. Clauditz TS, Reiff M, Gravert L, et al. Human epidermal growth factor receptor 2 (HER2) in salivary gland carcinomas. Pathology 2011;43(5):459–64.

20. Haddad R, Colevas AD, Krane JF, et al. Herceptin in patients with advanced or metastatic salivary gland carcinomas. A phase II study. Oral Oncol 2003;39(7): 724–7.

21. Thorpe LM, Schrock AB, Erlich RL, et al. Significant and durable clinical benefit from trastuzumab in 2 patients with HER2-amplified salivary gland cancer and a review of the literature. Head Neck 2017;39(3):E40–4.

22. Park JC, Ma TM, Rooper L, et al. Exceptional responses to pertuzumab, trastuzumab, and docetaxel in human epidermal growth factor receptor-2 high expressing salivary duct carcinomas. Head Neck 2018;40(12):E100–6.

23. Hanna GJ, Bae JE, Lorch JH, et al. The benefits of adjuvant trastuzumab for HER-2-positive salivary gland cancers. Oncologist 2020;25(7):598–608.

24. Takahashi H, Tada Y, Saotome T, et al. Phase II trial of trastuzumab and docetaxel in patients with human epidermal growth factor receptor 2-positive salivary duct carcinoma. J Clin Oncol 2019;37(2):125–34.

25. Kurzrock R, Bowles DW, Kang H, et al. Targeted therapy for advanced salivary gland carcinoma based on molecular profiling: results from MyPathway, a phase IIa multiple basket study. Ann Oncol 2020;31(3):412–21.

26. Chen S, Liang Y, Feng Z, et al. Efficacy and safety of HER2 inhibitors in combination with or without pertuzumab for HER2-positive breast cancer: a systematic review and meta-analysis. BMC Cancer 2019;19(1):973.

27. Li BT, Shen R, Offin M, et al. Ado-trastuzumab emtansine in patients with HER2 amplified salivary gland cancers (SGCs): results from a phase II basket trial. J Clin Oncol 2019;37(15_suppl):6001.

28. Shibuya M. Vascular endothelial growth factor (VEGF) and its receptor (VEGFR) signaling in angiogenesis: a crucial target for anti- and pro-angiogenic therapies. Genes Cancer 2011;2(12):1097–105.

29. Park S, Nam SJ, Keam B, et al. VEGF and Ki-67 overexpression in predicting poor overall survival in adenoid cystic carcinoma. Cancer Res Treat 2016;48(2): 518–26.

30. Hu-Lowe DD, Zou HY, Grazzini ML, et al. Nonclinical antiangiogenesis and anti-tumor activities of axitinib (AG-013736), an oral, potent, and selective inhibitor of vascular endothelial growth factor receptor tyrosine kinases 1, 2, 3. Clin Cancer Res 2008;14(22):7272–83.

31. Ho AL, Dunn L, Sherman EJ, et al. A phase II study of axitinib (AG-013736) in patients with incurable adenoid cystic carcinoma. Ann Oncol 2016;27(10):1902–8.

32. Locati LD, Cavalieri S, Bergamini C, et al. Phase II trial with axitinib in recurrent and/or metastatic salivary gland cancers of the upper aerodigestive tract. Head Neck 2019;41(10):3670–6.

33. Keam B, Kang EJ, Ahn M-J, et al. Randomized phase II study of axitinib versus observation in patients with recurred or metastatic adenoid cystic carcinoma. J Clin Oncol 2020;38(15_suppl):6503.

34. Kim Y, Lee SJ, Lee JY, et al. Clinical trial of nintedanib in patients with recurrent or metastatic salivary gland cancer of the head and neck: a multicenter phase 2 study (Korean Cancer Study Group HN14-01). Cancer 2017;123(11):1958–64.

35. Zhu G, Zhang L, Li R, et al. Phase II trial of apatinib in patients with recurrent and/or metastatic adenoid cystic carcinoma of the head and neck: Updated analysis. J Clin Oncol 2018;36(15_suppl):6026.

36. Stephens PJ, Davies HR, Mitani Y, et al. Whole exome sequencing of adenoid cystic carcinoma. J Clin Invest 2013;123(7):2965–8.

37. Miglarese MR, Halaban R, Gibson NW. Regulation of fibroblast growth factor 2 expression in melanoma cells by the c-MYB proto-oncoprotein. Cell Growth Differ 1997;8(11):1199–210.

38. Lee SH, Lopes de Menezes D, Vora J, et al. In vivo target modulation and biological activity of CHIR-258, a multitargeted growth factor receptor kinase inhibitor, in colon cancer models. Clin Cancer Res 2005;11(10):3633–41.

39. Keam B, Kim SB, Shin SH, et al. Phase 2 study of dovitinib in patients with metastatic or unresectable adenoid cystic carcinoma. Cancer 2015;121(15):2612–7.

40. Dillon PM, Petroni GR, Horton BJ, et al. A phase II study of dovitinib in patients with recurrent or metastatic adenoid cystic carcinoma. Clin Cancer Res 2017; 23(15):4138–45.

41. Wilhelm SM, Adnane L, Newell P, et al. Preclinical overview of sorafenib, a multi-kinase inhibitor that targets both Raf and VEGF and PDGF receptor tyrosine kinase signaling. Mol Cancer Ther 2008;7(10):3129–40.

42. Thomson DJ, Silva P, Denton K, et al. Phase II trial of sorafenib in advanced salivary adenoid cystic carcinoma of the head and neck. Head Neck 2015;37(2): 182–7.

43. Locati LD, Perrone F, Cortelazzi B, et al. A phase II study of sorafenib in recurrent and/or metastatic salivary gland carcinomas: translational analyses and clinical impact. Eur J Cancer 2016;69:158–65.

44. Chau NG, Hotte SJ, Chen EX, et al. A phase II study of sunitinib in recurrent and/or metastatic adenoid cystic carcinoma (ACC) of the salivary glands: current progress and challenges in evaluating molecularly targeted agents in ACC. Ann Oncol 2012;23(6):1562–70.

45. Hao Z, Wang P. Lenvatinib in management of solid tumors. Oncologist 2020; 25(2):e302–10.

46. Tchekmedyian V, Sherman EJ, Dunn L, et al. Phase II study of lenvatinib in patients with progressive, recurrent or metastatic adenoid cystic carcinoma. J Clin Oncol 2019;37(18):1529–37.

47. Skálová A, Vanecek T, Sima R, et al. Mammary analogue secretory carcinoma of salivary glands, containing the ETV6-NTRK3 fusion gene: a hitherto undescribed salivary gland tumor entity. Am J Surg Pathol 2010;34(5):599–608.

48. Cocco E, Scaltriti M, Drilon A. NTRK fusion-positive cancers and TRK inhibitor therapy. Nat Rev Clin Oncol 2018;15(12):731–47.

49. Drilon A, Siena S, Ou SI, et al. Safety and antitumor activity of the multitargeted Pan-TRK, ROS1, and ALK inhibitor entrectinib: combined results from two phase I trials (ALKA-372-001 and STARTRK-1). Cancer Discov 2017;7(4):400–9.

50. Drilon A, Laetsch TW, Kummar S, et al. Efficacy of Larotrectinib in TRK fusion-positive cancers in adults and children. N Engl J Med 2018;378(8):731–9.

51. Zarif JC, Miranti CK. The importance of non-nuclear AR signaling in prostate cancer progression and therapeutic resistance. Cell Signal 2016;28(5):348–56.

52. Williams MD, Roberts D, Blumenschein GR Jr, et al. Differential expression of hormonal and growth factor receptors in salivary duct carcinomas: biologic significance and potential role in therapeutic stratification of patients. Am J Surg Pathol 2007;31(11):1645–52.

53. Dalin MG, Watson PA, Ho AL, et al. Androgen receptor signaling in salivary gland cancer. Cancers (Basel) 2017;9(2):17.

54. Kamata YU, Sumida T, Murase R, et al. Blockade of androgen-induced malignant phenotypes by flutamide administration in human salivary duct carcinoma cells. Anticancer Res 2016;36(11):6071–5.

55. Yamamoto N, Minami S, Fujii M. Clinicopathologic study of salivary duct carcinoma and the efficacy of androgen deprivation therapy. Am J Otol 2014;35(6):731–5.

56. Poxleitner P, Shoumariyeh K, Steybe D, et al. Combined androgen deprivation therapy in recurrent androgen-receptor-positive salivary duct carcinoma - a case report and review of the literature. J Stomatol Oral Maxillofac Surg 2020;121(5):599–603.

57. Boon E, van Boxtel W, Buter J, et al. Androgen deprivation therapy for androgen receptor-positive advanced salivary duct carcinoma: a nationwide case series of 35 patients in The Netherlands. Head Neck 2018;40(3):605–13.

58. van Boxtel W, Verhaegh GW, van Engen-van Grunsven IA, et al. Prediction of clinical benefit from androgen deprivation therapy in salivary duct carcinoma patients. Int J Cancer 2020;146(11):3196–206.

59. Viscuse PV, Price KA, Garcia JJ, et al. First line androgen deprivation therapy vs. Chemotherapy for patients with androgen receptor positive recurrent or metastatic salivary gland carcinoma-a retrospective study. Front Oncol 2019;9:701.

60. Fushimi C, Tada Y, Takahashi H, et al. A prospective phase II study of combined androgen blockade in patients with androgen receptor-positive metastatic or locally advanced unresectable salivary gland carcinoma. Ann Oncol 2018;29(4):979–84.

61. Ho AL, Foster NR, Zoroufy AJ, et al. Alliance A091404: A phase II study of enzalutamide (NSC# 766085) for patients with androgen receptor-positive salivary cancers. J Clin Oncol 2019;37(15_suppl):6020.

62. van Boxtel W, Locati LD, van Engen-van Grunsven ACH, et al. Adjuvant androgen deprivation therapy for poor-risk, androgen receptor-positive salivary duct carcinoma. Eur J Cancer 2019;110:62–70.

63. Su BH, Qu J, Song M, et al. NOTCH1 signaling contributes to cell growth, anti-apoptosis and metastasis in salivary adenoid cystic carcinoma. Oncotarget 2014;5(16):6885–95.

64. Ferrarotto R, Mitani Y, Diao L, et al. Activating NOTCH1 mutations define a distinct subgroup of patients with adenoid cystic carcinoma who have poor prognosis, propensity to bone and liver metastasis, and potential responsiveness to notch1 inhibitors. J Clin Oncol 2017;35(3):352–60.

65. Chen W, Cao G, Yuan X, et al. Notch-1 knockdown suppresses proliferation, migration and metastasis of salivary adenoid cystic carcinoma cells. J Transl Med 2015;13:167.

66. Even C, Lassen U, Merchan J, et al. Safety and clinical activity of the Notch inhibitor, crenigacestat (LY3039478), in an open-label phase I trial expansion cohort of advanced or metastatic adenoid cystic carcinoma. Invest New Drugs 2020;38(2): 402–9.

67. Ferrarotto R, Wirth LJ, Muzaffar J, Rodriguez CP, Xia B, Perez CA, Bowles DW, Winquist E, Hotte SJ, Metcalf R, Even C, Gordon GB, Gordon G, Ho A. Annals of Oncology 2020; 31(suppl_4):s599-S628.

68. Zandberg DP, Strome SE. The role of the PD-L1:PD-1 pathway in squamous cell carcinoma of the head and neck. Oral Oncol 2014;50(7):627–32.

69. Mukaigawa T, Hayashi R, Hashimoto K, et al. Programmed death ligand-1 expression is associated with poor disease free survival in salivary gland carcinomas. J Surg Oncol 2016;114(1):36–43.

70. Theocharis S, Tasoulas J, Masaoutis C, et al. Salivary gland cancer in the era of immunotherapy: can we exploit tumor microenvironment? Expert Opin Ther Targets 2020;1–13. https://doi.org/10.1080/14728222.2020.1804863.

71. Cohen RB, Delord JP, Doi T, et al. Pembrolizumab for the treatment of advanced salivary gland carcinoma: findings of the phase 1b KEYNOTE-028 study. Am J Clin Oncol 2018;41(11):1083–8.

72. Fessas P, Lee H, Ikemizu S, et al. A molecular and preclinical comparison of the PD-1-targeted T-cell checkpoint inhibitors nivolumab and pembrolizumab. Semin Oncol 2017;44(2):136–40.

73. Fayette J, Even C, Digue L, et al. NISCAHN: A phase II, multicenter nonrandomized trial aiming at evaluating nivolumab (N) in two cohorts of patients (pts) with recurrent/metastatic (R/M) salivary gland carcinoma of the head and neck (SGCHN), on behalf of the Unicancer Head & Neck Group. J Clin Oncol 2019; 37(15_suppl):6083.

74. Chae YK, Othus M, Patel SP, et al. Abstract 3418: A phase II basket trial of dual anti-CTLA-4 and anti-PD-1 blockade in rare tumors (DART) SWOG S1609: The salivary gland tumor cohort. Cancer Res 2020;80(16 Supplement):3418.

75. Woods DM, Sodré AL, Villagra A, et al. HDAC inhibition upregulates PD-1 ligands in melanoma and augments immunotherapy with PD-1 Blockade. Cancer Immunol Res 2015;3(12):1375–85.

76. Johnstone RW. Histone-deacetylase inhibitors: novel drugs for the treatment of cancer. Nat Rev Drug Discov 2002;1(4):287–99.

77. Rodriguez CP, Wu QV, Voutsinas J, et al. A phase II trial of pembrolizumab and vorinostat in recurrent metastatic head and neck squamous cell carcinomas and salivary gland cancer. Clin Cancer Res 2020;26(4):837–45.

78. Goncalves PH, Heilbrun LK, Barrett MT, et al. A phase 2 study of vorinostat in locally advanced, recurrent, or metastatic adenoid cystic carcinoma. Oncotarget 2017;8(20):32918–29.

The Evaluation and Management of Carcinoma of the Minor Salivary Glands

Rohan Walvekar, MD*, Neelam Prakash Phalke, MD

KEYWORDS

- Minor salivary gland • Salivary gland carcinoma • Mucoepidermoid carcinoma
- Adenoid cystic carcinoma

KEY POINTS

- The minor salivary glands are located throughout the upper aerodigestive tract.
- Salivary gland carcinomas are a rare malignancy affecting the head and neck accounting for less than 3% of all head and neck malignancies. Of malignant tumors of the salivary glands, less than 15% are in the minor glands.
- Compared with the major salivary glands masses, which tend to be benign, about 80% of all tumors of the minor glands are malignant.
- Minor salivary gland malignancies are often detected late because of the location, and the fact that they are not capsulated may influence their invasive potential into adjacent tissues.
- Adequate surgical resection of minor salivary gland tumors, even when higher grade malignancy, has the potential to yield 5-year survival rates of greater 70%.

INTRODUCTION

The salivary glands are secretory glands located in the head and neck that produce saliva and release it into the oral cavity via ductal systems (**Table 1**). Saliva functions as a lubricant for the protection of oral cavity structures and in the clearance and digestion of food. There are three major paired glands: (1) parotids, (2) submandibular glands, and (3) sublingual glands. There are approximately 400 to 700 minor salivary glands located throughout the upper aerodigestive tract. The minor salivary glands function similarly to the major glands. The minor salivary glands are affected by similar pathologies from infection and dysfunction to tumor growth. In contrast to the major salivary glands, in which benign tumors are more common, the likelihood of a tumor of the minor salivary glands being benign or malignant is nearly equivalent. This review

Department of Otolaryngology–Head & Neck Surgery, Louisiana State University Health Sciences Campus, 533 Bolivar Street, Suite 566, New Orleans, LA 70112, USA
* Corresponding author.
E-mail address: rwalve@lsuhsc.edu

Otolaryngol Clin N Am 54 (2021) 629–639
https://doi.org/10.1016/j.otc.2021.02.011
0030-6665/21/© 2021 Elsevier Inc. All rights reserved.

oto.theclinics.com

Table 1
Staging of minor salivary gland carcinoma per American Joint Committee on Cancer 8th edition guidelines

T Stage	Size	Extent
T1	<2 cm	No extraparenchymal extension
T2	2–4 cm	
T3	>4 cm	Any extraparenchymal extension
T4a	Any size	Invasion of skin, mandible, external auditory canal, or facial nerve
T4b		Invasion of skull base or pterygoid plates; or encasement of the carotid artery

focuses on the identification and management malignant neoplasms that affect these minor salivary glands.

ANATOMY AND PHYSIOLOGY

The minor salivary glands develop during the twelfth week of gestation from the ectoderm of the oral cavity and nasopharynx. They are mainly concentrated into four regions: (1) buccal, (2) labial, (3) palatal, and (4) lingual. They are unencapsulated glands that are typically submucosal in location but are found within the oropharyngeal musculature.[1] Blood supply to the minor salivary glands comes from regional vasculature. The minor salivary glands receive postganglionic parasympathetic fibers from the submandibular ganglion. The only exception are the palatine minor salivary glands, which are innervated by postganglionic parasympathetic fibers from the sphenopalatine ganglion.

Each salivary gland is composed of secretory units made of acinar cells and myoepithelial cells. The ductal systems are made of epithelial cells. The functional cells of the salivary glands are the acinar cells. There are three types of acinar cells: (1) serous cells that secrete a waterier saliva; (2) mucus cells that secrete a thicker, mucoid saliva; and (3) mixed cells that secrete saliva with mixed characteristics. The myoepithelial cells function to help move the acinar cell secretions into the ductal system and then into the oral cavity. The major function, then, of the minor salivary glands is the production of saliva, a lubricant that also has antimicrobial protective properties.[1]

EPIDEMIOLOGY

Salivary gland neoplasms are fairly uncommon with a reported incidence of 0.4 to 2.6 per 100,000 people. They occur typically in the sixth to seventh decade of life and have a slightly higher incidence in men than women. Most salivary neoplasms occur in the parotid glands. Eighty percent are found to be benign. By contrast, 80% of minor salivary gland neoplasms tend to be malignant. Overall, salivary gland carcinoma represents less than 3% of all head and neck malignancies,[2–4] of which only 10% to 15% are from the minor glands.[5]

The pathologies affecting minor salivary glands are the same as those affecting the major glands. The most common benign neoplasm is the pleomorphic adenoma. Of malignant tumors found in the minor salivary glands, the most common are mucoepidermoid carcinoma (39%–40%), adenoid cystic carcinoma (24%–31%), and polymorphous low-grade adenocarcinoma (PLGA) (12%–24%).[6,7] The most common site of minor salivary gland tumor is the soft palate, followed by the nasal cavity, and then the tongue.[8,9]

Common benign and malignant pathologies identified in a large study of minor salivary glands tumors are listed next in order of most frequent to least[10]:

Benign
- Pleomorphic adenoma
- Basal cell adenoma
- Cystadenoma
- Myoepithelioma
- Oncocytoma
- Sialadenoma papilliferum

Malignant
- Mucoepidermoid carcinoma
- Adenoid cystic carcinoma
- PLGA
- Adenocarcinoma not specified
- Basal cell adenocarcinoma
- Clear cell carcinoma
- Salivary ductal carcinoma
- Carcinoma ex pleomorphic adenoma
- Mucinous adenocarcinoma
- Sebaceous carcinoma

RISK FACTORS FOR SALIVARY GLAND CARCINOMA INCLUDE

- Tobacco use
- Alcohol use
- History of radiation to the head and neck
- History of any cancer
- Human immunodeficiency virus (HIV) infection

Protective factors may be related to diet.[2,3,8] Vitamin C and fiber from fruit and vegetable sources have been found to lower the risk of salivary gland cancer. Diets high in cholesterol are associated with increased risk.[3]

PRESENTATION

Patients typically present with asymptomatic, painless swelling or mass. Patients presenting later in their disease course may have pain. It must be borne in mind that pain at presentation is a red flag for a perineural invasion associated with malignant tumors or malignant conversion in a benign tumor. In patients who do present with symptomatic masses, their symptoms tend to be related to mass effect or infiltration of adjacent structures. Minor salivary gland carcinoma of the sinonasal cavity can present with epistaxis or nasal obstruction. In the oropharynx and larynx, masses may result in dysphagia, dysphonia, or dyspnea. Physical examination may reveal a submucosal mass with adherent mucosa with or without overlying ulceration (**Fig. 1**).[2,11,12]

The differential diagnosis for this presentation includes acute necrotizing sialometaplasia, mucocele, and mucus retention cysts.[1,13]

Acute Necrotizing Sialometaplasia

This is a benign lesion most commonly seen on the palate. The lesion presents as a painful mass that eventually ulcerates. In this early stage, these lesions can look similar to basal cell carcinomas or other neoplasms with rolled edges over a central ulceration. As this disease process progresses, the lesion mucosalizes and heals over a

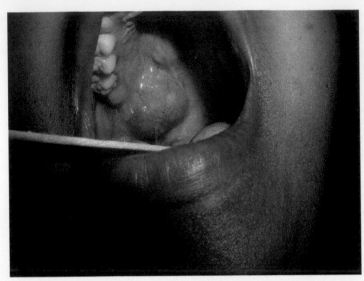

Fig. 1. Patient with enlarging hard palatal mass found to be adenoid cystic carcinoma. (*Courtesy of* Dr. Boyd Gillespie.)

period of several weeks. However, most tumors are often biopsied and/or surgically excised before this stage because of their concerning clinical presentation and appearance. On pathologic evaluation, the squamous metaplasia can appear similar to mucoepidermoid carcinoma.

Mucocele

Mucoceles present as a painless or painful oral submucosal mass. They typically occur after trauma that results in injury to the salivary duct and are characterized by submucosal accumulation of saliva with surrounding inflammation and granulation tissue without a true epithelial capsule.

Mucus Retention Cyst

These also present as a painless oral mass and result from an obstruction of a salivary duct resulting in mucoid salivary accumulation. Unlike mucoceles, mucus retention cysts they have a capsule lined by ductal epithelium. They more commonly affect the major salivary glands.

OTHER LESS COMMON PATHOLOGIES INCLUDE

- Lymphoepithelial cysts (see most commonly in HIV patients)
- Metastatic cutaneous malignancy, especially melanoma
- Benign masses, including epidermoid cysts, fibromas, and bony tori of the mandible or hard palate

IMAGING

Imaging is used to further characterize size and extent of the tumor. Initial imaging may involve ultrasound to characterize the nature of the mass (solid, cystic, or mixed) and location (intraglandular or extraglandular). For more definitive imaging, MRI is preferred over computed tomography (CT) in the case of minor salivary glands given their size and the need to define tumor from surrounding soft and neural tissues. Precontrast and postcontrast MRIs are used to identify perineural spread, especially along the palatine nerves for palatal masses. MRI can also be used to differentiate between benign and malignant masses. On T2-weighted imaging, benign masses tend to be hyperintense, whereas malignant masses are hypointense. CT is complementary to MRI and helps with determination of bony erosion or invasion. Finally, PET scanning should be performed in cases of confirmed malignancy to rule out regional disease and systemic metastasis (**Figs. 2–4**).[2,14,15]

DIAGNOSIS

Tissue diagnosis is usually obtained through fine-needle aspiration, which has a sensitivity and a specificity of 87% to 96%.[16] Incisional biopsy is not routinely recommended because it can result in tumor violation and possibly impact recurrence potential.[17] However, the value of obtaining a diagnosis before surgical intervention is important for planning of surgical margins, extent of surgery, and reconstruction. Consequently, depending on the clinical presentation, site of tumor, and access, a biopsy can be obtained either through methods described previously, such as ultrasound-guided fine-needle aspiration, or core biopsy, incisional biopsy, or an excisional biopsy. Preoperative planning with imaging allows identification of nearby nerves and vasculature that may be at risk for injury during resection or that may need to be resected based on tumor proximity or obvious involvement (**Fig. 5**).

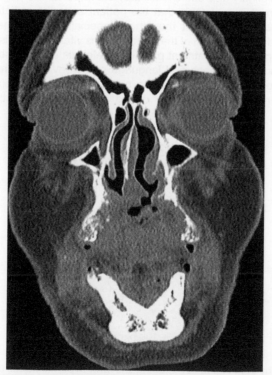

Fig. 2. A 74-year-old man with mucoepidermoid carcinoma of a hard palate minor salivary gland. CT without contrast showing destructive lesion of the anterior maxilla.

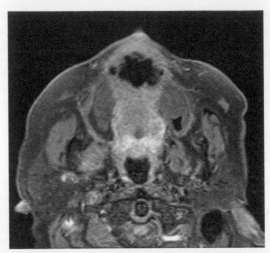

Fig. 3. Same patient as in **Fig. 2**. T2 fat-suppressed MRI showing oronasal fistula secondary to destructive lesion of the hard palate.

INVOLVEMENT OF THE HEALTH CARE TEAM

As with all malignancy, management of patients with salivary gland carcinoma involves a multidisciplinary approach; therefore, it is important to begin involving other providers early on. It is preferable that the patient sees the radiation and medical oncologist preoperatively so that they these specialists have the opportunity to make an independent evaluation of the tumor. This is vital for multidisciplinary discussions, tumor mapping, and treatment planning. Referrals should also include rehabilitative services, such as speech and language pathology for pretreatment swallow evaluation and post-treatment therapy; to nutrition to ensure adequate intake and supplementation recommendations for during and after treatment; to dentistry for

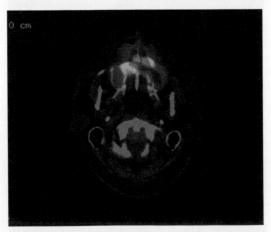

Fig. 4. Same patient as in **Fig. 2**. PET imaging showing hypermetabolic uptake at the hard palate and maxilla alveolar ridge at the site of the fistula with maximum standardized uptake value of 14.2.

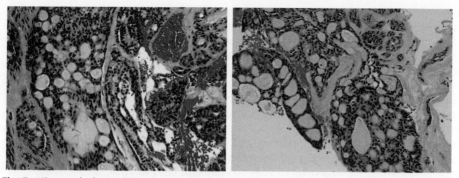

Fig. 5. Histopathologic slides depicting adenoid cystic carcinoma of the soft palate from the case in **Fig. 2**. (*Courtesy of* Tracy Rauch, MD, Baton Rouge, LA.)

dental extractions, especially in patients undergoing radiation therapy; and, where available and appropriate, to psychology or counseling services. Assessment of patient's social situation and planning transportation, disposition, and financial considerations are an important part of the overall treatment experience and impact efficiency of care.

MANAGEMENT

The mainstay of therapy for minor salivary gland carcinoma is surgical resection with or without adjuvant radiation based on grade and staging of the tumor. If the surgical margins involve bony resection (ie, the maxilla or mandible) adequate consideration must be given to appropriate reconstruction; in most scenarios a free tissue transfer is necessary and is usually performed at the time of surgical excision.[9] Lymph node dissection is based on clinical and/or radiographic findings of suspicious nodes or grade of the tumor.[2,8] For node-negative necks, elective neck dissection is dependent on the histologic type of the tumor, as is described while discussing individual pathologic types. Neck irradiation is an option for the management of occult metastasis in clinically node-negative necks, especially when malignant pathology is discovered incidentally after surgical management of a minor salivary gland neoplasm.[18,19] When indicated for management, a selective dissection of relevant nodal basin for the location of the primary (eg, I-IV or I-III) is performed.[20]

Radiation alone is not routinely recommended for primary management of minor salivary gland malignancies because it tends to have inferior long-term survival rates. A study of all types and locations of minor salivary gland cancer by Salgado and colleagues[21] looked at radiation outcomes in terms of local and distant control. Local control was only 87.9% at 5 years and 80.5% at 10 years. The rates of distant metastasis were 17% at 5 years and 37% at 10 years.[21]

Local recurrence is not uncommon with salivary gland malignancies. Distant metastases are most commonly to the lungs. As such, all patients with any minor salivary gland carcinoma require long-term follow-up.[2,20] Recurrence is managed similarly with surgery and/or reirradiation. The goal of management for recurrence may be local tumor control or palliation.[2,8]

Mucoepidermoid Carcinoma

Mucoepidermoid carcinoma arising from the mucus and epidermal cells of salivary glands is categorized into low-grade or high-grade types based on cell types.

Low-grade tumors feature more mucous cells, whereas high-grade tumors are dominated by squamous cells with significant atypia similar in appearance to squamous cell carcinoma. More recently, there has been the delineation of intermediate-grade tumors that are formed of sheets of squamous cells but retain a more cystic-like structure similar to low-grade tumors.[22]

Low-grade tumors are managed with wide local resection only. Neck dissection and adjuvant radiation are not indicated.[20] High-grade tumors tend to be locally invasive and also have a significant potential for regional metastasis with an occult rate of metastasis being 21%. Consequently, high-grade minor salivary gland carcinomas are managed with surgical resection and neck dissection or adjuvant therapy (for occult local metastasis). Long-term survival is generally good with overall 5- and 10-year disease-free survival rates of 75% to 78% and 68% to 75%, respectively.[6,23]

Adenoid Cystic Carcinoma

Adenoid cystic carcinoma arises from the epithelial and myoepithelial cells of the salivary glands. The tumor tends to be infiltrative at presentation. Although it is slow growing, it has a strong propensity for distant metastasis, even more so than local metastasis. Late distant metastasis is a distinguishing feature of adenoid cystic carcinoma that contributes to its lower long-term survival rates.[24] There are three histologic types (cribriform, tubular, and solid), with solid having the worst prognosis.

Management requires complete surgical excision and adjuvant radiation. Occult regional lymph node metastasis is uncommon, so elective neck dissection is not recommended routinely.[20] Furthermore, studies have shown that prognostic outcome for adenoid cystic carcinoma is not significantly changed by the involvement of local nodes at time of diagnosis.[12] However, similar to mucoepidermoid carcinoma, many authors argue for postoperative neck irradiation for protection against occult metastasis.[18,19] Mortality from adenoid cystic carcinoma is typically related to distant metastasis with 5- and 10-year survival rates of 68% to 79% and 37% to 63%, respectively.[6,23]

Polymorphous Low-Grade Adenocarcinoma

PLGA is a rare tumor that uniquely tends to affect minor salivary glands, although it can occur in the major glands. It is most commonly seen in palatal minor glands. Like other adenocarcinomas, this tumor arises from the mucus-secreting acinar cells of the salivary glands. The cells grow in uniform single-layer strands that form a variety of patterns. The most common are tubular, solid, and papillary; however, there have been other well-characterized patterns found, such as microcystic or cribriform. A clear association between pattern type and prognosis has not yet been well defined.[25–27]

PLGAs are considered low grade because they tend to be slow growing with lower rates of metastasis compared with other minor salivary gland malignancies. As such, management is based on primary local control with wide surgical excision. Adjuvant radiation is not usually necessary. Local metastasis occurs at a rate of 5% to 15%; therefore, elective neck dissection is not routinely recommended. A review of patients diagnosed and treated for PLGA of the head and neck in the SEER database by Patel and colleagues[26] supports this recommendation. Of 460 cases, 322 underwent surgical resection alone. Of those only 15 patients without clinical evidence of nodal disease underwent elective neck dissection; 94.7% did not undergo any neck dissection. The 5-year disease-free survival rate for the entire population (including the 5.3% who underwent elective neck dissection) was 99.3%.[26,27]

LONG-TERM OUTCOMES

In general, tumor of the oral cavity, especially palatal minor salivary gland carcinomas, have the best outcomes.[28] Sinonasal tumors and minor salivary gland carcinomas have the worst prognosis, regardless of histologic type. The 5-year survival rates for minor salivary gland carcinomas found in the oral cavity, oropharynx, and sinonasal cavities are around 84% to 89%. However, at 10 years, the survival rate is 74% for oral cavity tumors and drops to 59% for oropharyngeal tumors and 57% for sinonasal tumors.[7]

Based on final pathologic staging, the 5- and 10-year overall survival rates are as follows: for T1 tumors, 92% and 82%; for T2 tumors, 82% and 60%; for T3 tumors, 95% with a significant drop in survival to 24%; and for T4 tumors, 73% and 53%. Of note is the more severe drop in survival at 10 years in the T3 group compared with the T4 group. Hay and colleagues[7] comment this is likely the result of a smaller sample size for the T3 population given the inability of a tumor in the oropharyngeal space to get very large without invasion of major structures, necessitating upstaging. With nodal involvement the 5-year survival rate drops from 90% for N0 to 62% to 67% for N1 and N2. At 10 years for pathologically node-positive disease the survival rate is 33% to 40%.[7]

The overall survival rates based on all histologic subtypes of minor salivary gland carcinomas are 66% and 57% at 5- and 10-years, respectively. Disease-free survival ranges from 48% to 68% at 5 years and 37% to 68% at 10 years. However, the survival between 5 and 10 years for mucoepidermoid carcinoma and PLGA is stable. Adenoid cystic carcinoma tends to present with late distant metastasis and there is a considerable drop in survival between the 5- and 10-year marks.[6,11,20,29]

SUMMARY

Minor salivary glands are widely present throughout the upper aerodigestive tract, but tumors of these glands are an uncommon pathology of the head and neck. Minor salivary gland neoplasms have a high malignant potential; consequently, it is imperative to maintain a high level of suspicion when a concerning lesion is identified. Management is essentially surgical with adjuvant therapy when indicated resulting in good long-term survival rates for early stage tumors. A multimodality approach is required for advanced-stage tumors wherein primary nonsurgical therapy is a viable option for patients who have technically unresectable disease or do not want to opt for surgical management.

CLINICS CARE POINTS

- A high level of suspicion should be maintained for lesions of the aerodigestive tract to rule out minor salivary gland neoplasm given the high rate of malignancy in tumors of these glands.
- Any concerning lesions should undergo biopsy for definitive tissue diagnosis.
- The gold standard for imaging of the minor salivary glands is MRI to determine size and perineural involvement. CT and PET scanning can also be performed to evaluate for bony erosion and metastasis.
- Management of any stage or histologic type is primarily based on surgical excision with or without adjuvant radiation.

- The most common histologic types are mucoepidermoid carcinoma and adenoid cystic carcinoma. These can be locally aggressive but have good 5-year disease-free survival rates with appropriate surgical and radiation treatments.

- Neck dissection at time of surgical resection is indicated for node-positive disease and could be an alternative to neck irradiation for a clinically negative neck.

- The role of postoperative adjuvant radiation is to manage occult local metastasis in patients who are clinically free of nodal disease and for whom elective neck dissection is not planned.

- The decision on elective neck dissection or elective neck irradiation is multifactorial and depends on clinical presentation, tumor site, histology, and patient factors; consequently, indication for neck dissection is best discussed in a multidisciplinary setting and personalized to each patient's unique presentation and circumstances.

- These tumors are associated with high local recurrence rates; thus, long-term follow-up is imperative to allow early diagnosis and treatment of recurrence.

DISCLOSURE

Nothing to disclose.

REFERENCES

1. Aframian DJ, Keshet N, Nadler C, et al. Minor salivary glands: clinical, histological and immunohistochemical features of common and less common pathologies. Acta Histochem 2019;121(8):151451.
2. Guzzo M, Locati LD, Prott FJ, et al. Major and minor salivary gland tumors. Crit Rev Oncol Hematol 2010;74(2):134–48.
3. Horn-Ross PL, Morrow M, Ljung BM. Diet and the risk of salivary gland cancer. Am J Epidemiol 1997;146(2):171–6.
4. Wang X-d, Meng L-j, Hou T-t, et al. Tumours of the salivary glands in northeastern China: a retrospective study of 2508 patients. Br J Oral Maxillofac Surg 2015; 53(2):132–7.
5. Vander Poorten V, Hunt J, Bradley PJ, et al. Recent trends in the management of minor salivary gland carcinoma. Head Neck 2014;36(3):444–55.
6. Iyer NG, Kim L, Nixon IJ, et al. Factors predicting outcome in malignant minor salivary gland tumors of the oropharynx. Arch Otolaryngol Head Neck Surg 2010;136(12):1240–7.
7. Hay AJ, Migliacci J, Karassawa Zanoni D, et al. Minor salivary gland tumors of the head and neck-Memorial Sloan Kettering experience: incidence and outcomes by site and histological type. Cancer 2019;125(19):3354–66.
8. Licitra L, Grandi C, Prott FJ, et al. Major and minor salivary glands tumours. Crit Rev Oncol Hematol 2003;45(2):215–25.
9. Carlson ER, Schlieve T. Salivary gland malignancies. Oral Maxillofac Surg Clin North Am 2019;31(1):125–44.
10. Venkata V, Irulandy P. The frequency and distribution pattern of minor salivary gland tumors in a government dental teaching hospital, Chennai, India. Oral Surg Oral Med Oral Pathol Oral Radiol Endod 2011;111(1):e32–9.
11. Spiro RH. Salivary neoplasms: overview of a 35-year experience with 2,807 patients. Head Neck Surg 1986;8(3):177–84.
12. Bianchi B, Copelli C, Cocchi R, et al. Adenoid cystic carcinoma of intraoral minor salivary glands. Oral Oncol 2008;44(11):1026–31.

13. Mohan H, Tahlan A, Mundi I, et al. Non-neoplastic salivary gland lesions: a 15-year study. Eur Arch Otorhinolaryngol 2011;268(8):1187–90.
14. Abdel Razek AAK, Mukherji SK. Imaging of minor salivary glands. Neuroimaging Clin N Am 2018;28(2):295–302.
15. Sengupta A, Brown J, Rudralingam M. The use of intraoral ultrasound in the characterization of minor salivary gland malignancy: report of two cases. Dentomaxillofac Radiol 2016;45(4):20150354.
16. Gal R. Fine need aspiration of the salivary glands: a review. Oper Tech Otolaryngol Head Neck Surg 1996;7(4):323–6.
17. Wei S, Layfield LJ, LiVolsi VA, et al. Reporting of fine needle aspiration (FNA) specimens of salivary gland lesions: a comprehensive review. Diagn Cytopathol 2017;45(9):820–7.
18. Le QT, Birdwell S, Terris DJ, et al. Postoperative irradiation of minor salivary gland malignancies of the head and neck. Radiother Oncol 1999;52(2):165–71.
19. Garden AS, Weber RS, Ang KK, et al. Postoperative radiation therapy for malignant tumors of minor salivary glands. Outcome and patterns of failure. Cancer 1994;73(10):2563–9.
20. Lee SY, Shin HA, Rho KJ, et al. Characteristics, management of the neck, and oncological outcomes of malignant minor salivary gland tumours in the oral and sinonasal regions. Br J Oral Maxillofac Surg 2013;51(7):e142–7.
21. Salgado LR, Spratt DE, Riaz N, et al. Radiation therapy in the treatment of minor salivary gland tumors. Am J Clin Oncol 2014;37(5):492–7.
22. Triantafillidou K, Dimitrakopoulos J, Iordanidis F, et al. Mucoepidermoid carcinoma of minor salivary glands: a clinical study of 16 cases and review of the literature. Oral Dis 2006;12(4):364–70.
23. Copelli C, Bianchi B, Ferrari S, et al. Malignant tumors of intraoral minor salivary glands. Oral Oncol 2008;44(7):658–63.
24. van der Wal JE, Becking AG, Snow GB, et al. Distant metastases of adenoid cystic carcinoma of the salivary glands and the value of diagnostic examinations during follow-up. Head Neck 2002;24(8):779–83.
25. Evans HL, Luna MA. Polymorphous low-grade adenocarcinoma: a study of 40 cases with long-term follow up and an evaluation of the importance of papillary areas. Am J Surg Pathol 2000;24(10):1319–28.
26. Patel TD, Vazquez A, Marchiano E, et al. Polymorphous low-grade adenocarcinoma of the head and neck: a population-based study of 460 cases. Laryngoscope 2015;125(7):1644–9.
27. de Araujo VC, Passador-Santos F, Turssi C, et al. Polymorphous low-grade adenocarcinoma: an analysis of epidemiological studies and hints for pathologists. Diagn Pathol 2013;8:6.
28. AJCC. Staging head and neck cancers. AJCC cancer staging manual. 8th edition 2018.
29. Vander Poorten VL, Balm AJ, Hilgers FJ, et al. Stage as major long term outcome predictor in minor salivary gland carcinoma. Cancer 2000;89(6):1195 204.

Extent and Indications for Elective and Therapeutic Neck Dissection for Salivary Carcinoma

Alexandra E. Kejner, MD[a],*, Brianna N. Harris, MD[b,1]

KEYWORDS

- Salivary gland malignancy • Salivary carcinoma • Neck dissection
- Therapeutic neck dissection • Elective neck dissection

KEY POINTS

- Salivary gland carcinomas are more likely to spread to lymph nodes in cases of high-grade malignancy, advanced T stage, perineural invasion, and extraglandular extension.
- Minor salivary gland carcinomas tend to have more high-risk features.
- Elective neck dissection should include at least levels 2 to 3 for parotid malignancies and levels 1 to 3 for lesions occurring in the submandibular gland.
- Therapeutic neck dissection should include at least levels 2 to 4 for parotid malignancy, and 1 to 3 for oral cavity salivary gland malignancy barring radiologically positive disease in other levels.
- Further prospective data are needed to illuminate guidelines for rare histologic subtypes.

INTRODUCTION/BACKGROUND
Nature of the Problem

Salivary gland carcinomas (SGC) are relatively uncommon, occurring at a rate of about 2.5 to 3/100,000 people per year in the United States (**Box 1**). They make up only 3% to 6% of all head and neck tumors. Worldwide, the incidence ranges from 0.05 to 2/100,000 people.[1] The incidence of SGC is increasing as are the rates of regional metastases.[2] Metastases from SGC have been reported to be as high as 65%. Nodal disease has been shown to worsen disease-specific survival.[3] Therefore, having a clear understanding of the indication for neck dissection is increasingly relevant.

[a] Department of Otolaryngology–Head and Neck Surgery, University of Kentucky, Lexington, KY, USA; [b] Department of Otolaryngology–Head and Neck Surgery, Scripps Health
[1] Present address: 3590 Camino Del Rio North, Suite 103, San Diego, CA 92108.
* Corresponding author. 740 South Limestone Road, E300E Kentucky Clinic, Lexington, KY 40502.
E-mail address: Alexandra.kejner@uky.edu

Otolaryngol Clin N Am 54 (2021) 641–651
https://doi.org/10.1016/j.otc.2021.02.006
0030-6665/21/© 2021 Elsevier Inc. All rights reserved.

> **Box 1**
> **Predictors of occult lymph node metastases**
>
> Site: Oral cavity (tongue), nasopharynx
>
> High-grade histologic subtypes:
>   High-grade mucoepidermoid; adenoid cystic carcinoma
>   Salivary ductal carcinoma
>
> Aggressive subtype: Cribriform adenocarcinoma of the minor salivary gland
>
> T3/T4 primary
>
> Elderly
>
> Perineural invasion/facial paralysis
>
> Perilymphatic invasion
>
> Extraparenchymal extension
>
> Periparotid lymph nodes (preauricular or intraparotid)

Given the low incidence and wide heterogeneity of salivary gland tumors, no randomized controlled trials exist to guide treatment. Furthermore, current National Comprehensive Cancer Network guidelines recommend neck dissection in cN0 neck only for high-grade or T3/T4 tumors of the major salivary glands but do not give explicit guidance for tumors of the minor salivary glands (MiSG).[4] Elective nodal dissection remains somewhat controversial because it is often performed based on age, on tumor size/grade, on surgeon preference, or at the discretion of multidisciplinary tumor boards. Most of the available literature is limited by small cohorts, recent changes in classifications and subtypes, and primary site location.[3]

Data extrapolated from mucosal head and neck primary tumors suggest that if the risk of occult metastases is greater than 15% to 20%, an elective neck dissection (END) should be performed. The rate of occult neck metastases from primary salivary gland malignancies ranges between 11% and 35%, with varying incidence based on subsite and histopathology. High-grade histology, in particular, is significantly associated with risk of lymph node metastases. However, pathologic grade is often unknown until the salivary gland tumor has been removed which is important in medically frail individuals given the potential morbidity from reoperation.[5]

For SGC with clinical, pathologic, or radiologic evidence of metastasis, therapeutic neck dissection is indicated; however, the extent of neck dissection (which levels to include) also remains debated. Therefore, the authors sought to determine which neoplasms are associated with high rates of occult metastases requiring neck dissection and to what extent neck dissection should be performed based on the current level of evidence.

INCIDENCE OF TUMOR TYPE BY SITE
Major Salivary Glands

Parotid
Most salivary gland neoplasms occur in the parotid gland (>80%), 20% of which are malignant. The incidence of malignant tumors in the parotid specifically is approximately 0.5 to 3/100,000 persons per year worldwide (5% of all head and neck malignancies).[6,7] In the United States, the incidence has been increasing over xx time period.[2] The most common malignant neoplasms in the parotid are mucoepidermoid carcinoma (MEC) (30%–35%), adenoid cystic carcinoma (AdCC) (15%–18%),

carcinoma ex pleomorphic (13%), acinic cell carcinoma (ACC) (~10%), and adeno-carcinoma not otherwise specified (NOS) (~5%). The remaining types of malignancy account for less than 5% of tumors found in the parotid.[8]

Submandibular. Although tumors occur in the submandibular gland less frequently than in the parotid gland, there is a higher propensity toward malignancy (up to 50%). They account for 0.1% of all head and neck malignancies, with an average incidence of approximately 1/100,000 persons per year. The most common malignancies of the submandibular gland are AdCC (37%–45%), MEC (15%–18%), carcinoma ex pleomorphic (16%), and ACC (4%). Other less commonly seen malignancies include salivary ductal carcinoma, lymphoepithelial carcinoma, myoepithelial carcinoma, and adenocarcinoma NOS.[9]

Sublingual. Less than 1% of SGCs arise within the sublingual gland with Surveillance, Epidemiology, and End Results Program (SEER) data demonstrating 0.11/100,000 persons per year. However, 70% to 90% of neoplasms in the sublingual gland are malignant. AdCC (0.04% overall incidence rate) and MEC (0.05% overall incidence rate) are the 2 most common types. Other types have been reported as well, including adenocarcinoma, myoepithelial carcinoma, and polymorphous low-grade adenocarcinoma (PLGA); although these are limited to case series and thus an incident rate is difficult to calculate.[10]

Minor salivary glands

MiSG tumors can arise in the sinonasal cavity, oral cavity, pharynx, larynx, trachea, lungs, and middle ear cavity. Carcinomas arising in the minor salivary glands make up about 22% of all SGCs.[11] Unlike the major salivary glands, most salivary neoplasms in the MiSGs are malignant. Similar to the parotid, the most common types are MEC (35%), AdCC (15%), and PLGA (10%). Unlike the major glands, however, ACC is not commonly seen. Please refer to the prior article on The Evaluation and Management of Carcinoma of the Minor Salivary Glands for further details.

Sinonasal/nasopharyngeal. AdCC is the most common SGC found in this region, followed by MEC. A review of English literature demonstrated a total of 98 reported cases, of which 95% were found to be AdCC. Nasopharyngeal SGC has a 47% rate of occult metastasis.[5]

Oral cavity and oropharynx. The oral cavity contains between 450 and 750 MiSG. The oral cavity is the most common site for MiSG cancer. AdCC and MEC are the most frequently encountered (35% and 21%, respectively), followed by PLGA (14%), adenocarcinoma NOS (11.6%), carcinoma ex pleomorphic, and others.[12]

Larynx. Most MiSGs are in the subglottis and supraglottis. MiSG cancers make up less than 1% of all laryngeal malignancies. It is equally found in men and women. There is no association with smoking. They commonly present with hoarseness, dysphagia, and cough. AdCC is the most common pathologic diagnosis, followed by MEC.[13] Often these are not amenable to local surgery; thus, total laryngectomy is needed. As such, neck dissection may be performed for vascular access if free tissue transfer is required. However, there are limited data regarding neck metastases. Neck dissection does not appear to confer a survival benefit in the cN0 neck for SGCs of the larynx.

RATE OF OCCULT METASTASES BY TUMOR TYPE
Adenoid Cystic Carcinoma

Literature rates of occult metastases are 15.38%. Results of an SEER analysis including 3026 patients with AdCC demonstrated a decline in incidence between

1973 and 2007.[14] The 5- and 10-year overall survival (OS) estimates were 90.3% and 79.8%, respectively. AdCC has a slight female preponderance. Female sex is associated with slightly improved survival with AdCC. In a study of 1784 patients with AdCC, 923 patients (51.7%) had primary tumor location in the parotid.[15] In this series, 70.4% of patients with parotid AdCC also underwent a neck dissection with 19% having positive lymph nodes. Furthermore, nearly 75% of patients underwent adjuvant radiation treatment, with postoperative radiation conferring an improved OS regardless of T stage. Similarly, in a small Canadian series, 40% occurred in the parotid with risk of lymph node metastasis at 12%. Overall prognosis was excellent.[16]

In a National Cancer Database (NCDB) study of AdCC, 38.8% (693) occurred in the submandibular gland. The authors found that, although submandibular location generally portends a worse prognosis, in this cohort, there was no difference in OS between primary subsites and no difference in risk of occult metastases.[15] Although this is the most common submandibular and MiSG malignancy, the rate of lymph node metastasis for submandibular AdCC is rare (4%); thus, neck dissection is generally not indicated. The propensity for late metastases in this subtype is generally related to perineural spread (**Fig. 1**), with the lung being the most common site for distant metastases (for all sites, AdCC).[17]

Mucoepidermoid Carcinoma

MEC is the most common salivary gland malignancy. Its incidence has been increasing over the last decade, with an incidence of 3.08/100,000 people.[2] The OS, Disease-free survival (DFS), and rate of metastasis are related to the histologic grade of the tumor. The 5-year survival for low-grade versus high-grade tumors is 86% versus 22%, respectively. Similarly, the DFS is 80% versus 30% for low- versus high-grade tumors.[18] The rate of occult metastasis in low-grade mucoepidermoid is near 0%, whereas high grade has been reported to be as high as 35% to 45%.[5] Therefore, elective treatment of the neck in low-grade mucoepidermoid is not recommended. Locoregional recurrence for low-grade MEC is approximately 10% with a 5-

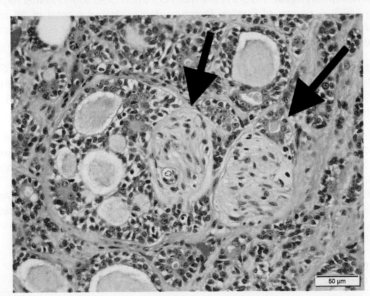

Fig. 1. AdCC. Tumor cells form cribriform structures and tubules. Arrows point to characteristic perineural invasion (H&E stain, x400).

year OS of 97%. For high-grade tumors, however, neck dissection is recommended at the time of the primary tumor resection, as occult metastases rates have been shown to be approximately 21%. Locoregional recurrence rates for high-grade MEC are significantly higher (43.5%) with a lower DFS. Therefore, in addition to neck dissection, adjuvant radiotherapy is often recommended.

Acinic cell carcinoma

AcCC is one of the most common salivary gland malignancies, behind MEC and AdCC, accounting for ~10% to 17% of all salivary gland cancers. Of these tumors, 98% occur in the parotid gland. Overall, AcCC has a less aggressive course and a good prognosis with a 90% 5-year survival and a 55% OS at 20 years.[19] The incidence of lymph node metastases in AcCC is approximately 10%, with a risk of occult disease occurring in up to 22% of cases.[19] In a study of 66 patients with AcCC of the parotid, 8 (12.1%) patients had clinical evidence of neck disease at presentation, and a therapeutic neck dissection was performed in all 8 patients. END was performed in 27 patients. Out of the 35 dissections performed, 12 (34.3%) were found to have pathologically positive nodes with occult nodes present in 4 patients (14.8%). Level II was the most common site of positive lymph nodes.[19] In another study of the NCDB, the rate of occult metastases in AcCC was 22%. Similarly, in a study of 144 patients, 22/31 (71%) cN+ patients had pathologic nodes, whereas 15/52 (28.9%) patients who underwent END had pathologic nodes. In this study, the extent of therapeutic and electives neck dissections were levels I to IV and I to III, respectively.[20] In general, END does not appear to be indicated, but in cases of advanced stage or presence of facial palsy, END can be considered.

Salivary ductal carcinoma

Salivary duct carcinoma is extremely rare (1%) but highly aggressive. Most of these tumors occur in the parotid gland (78%) but can also occur in the submandibular and MiSGs. Given their aggressive nature, more than 50% of these tumors present with cervical metastases at the time of diagnosis. Similarly, there is a high rate of local recurrence within 2 years of initial treatment. Similar to infiltrating ductal carcinoma of the breast, some tumors stain positive for HER2/neu. Positivity is associated with a poorer prognosis (<15% 5-year survival) (Fig 2A, B). Therefore, neck dissection and adjuvant therapy are recommended.

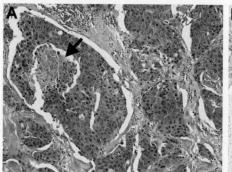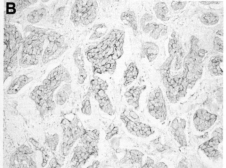

Fig. 2. Salivary duct carcinoma. (*A*) Tumor forms nests often with central necrosis (*arrow*) (H&E, x200). (*B*) Characteristic nuclear expression for androgen receptors; some tumors also show membranous reactivity for HER2 [Brown chromagen and hematoxylin counterstain; x200].

Carcinoma ex pleomorphic

Carcinoma ex pleomorphic represents 2% to 5% of all salivary gland tumors arising from a preexisting pleomorphic adenoma. Neurovascular invasion is relatively common in these tumors, as are local and distant metastases. Occult neck disease has been shown to be approximately 20%, with a recurrence rate around 30% to 35%. Nodal disease is a significant prognostic indicator of OS, with 1 study demonstrating

Table 1				
Salivary glands with pathologic condition types and occult metastases				
Salivary Glands	Pathology Types	Occult Metastases, %	Levels	End
Parotid	MEC (30%–35%)			
	Low	3.30		N
	Intermediate	8.10		N
	High	34	I-V[a]	Y
	AdCC (15%–18%)	14.5[b]	I-III	Y[c]
	AcCC (10%)	14.8[d]	See comment	Y[b]
	(<5%)	20	I-III	Y
	Other (5%)			
	Salivary ductal carcinoma	11.80	I-V	Y
	Lymphoepithelial/myoepithelial	<1		N
	Adenocarcinoma NOS	23.60	I-III	Y
Submandibular	AdCC (37%–45%)	21.3[b]	I-III[b]	Y
	MEC (15%–18%)	34	I-IV[a] (high grade only)	Y
	Carcinoma ex pleomorphic (16%)	20	Nil	Y
	AcCC (4%)	14.8[d]	See comment	Y[c]
	Other (5%)			
	Salivary ductal		I-IV	Y
	Lymphoepithelial/Myoepithelial	<1		
	Adenocarcinoma NOS	*High*	I-IV	Y
Sublingual	AdCC (80%)	24.70	I-III	Y
	MEC (9%)	ND	I-III (high grade only)	Y
	Adenocarcinoma NOS (11%}	ND	I-III	Y
Minor salivary				
OC/OP	AdCC	15–17	I-III	Y
	PLGA and CASMG	5–15[c]	I-III[c]	Y[c]
	Salivary ductal carcinoma	*High*	I-IV	Y
NP	AdCC/MEC	47	I-V	Y
Larynx	AdCC/MEC	<15		N

Abbreviations: N, no; ND, no data; Y, yes.

[a] 8.7% rate of skip metastases in high-grade MEC to level IV in parotid SGC.

[b] For adenoid cystic and AcCC, T stage was the most important factor with regard to occult metastases (T3 and T4 most likely to have occult metastases).

[c] For PLGA of the palate, low likelihood of metastasis. However, for extrapalatal OR cribriform/papillary histology, there is a significant risk of occult metastases and neck dissection is indicated.

[d] In general, if low-grade AcCC, END does not appear to be indicated, but in cases of advanced stage, presence of facial palsy, or high-grade tumors, END should be considered.

Data from Refs.[11,17,22–25]

the N+ disease had 5-year survival around 16%, versus 67% for N0 disease. Therefore, END is recommended in these cases.

Adenocarcinoma

Adenocarcinoma represents approximately 12% of salivary neoplasms and occurs in the MiSGs most commonly, followed by the parotid. They demonstrate aggressive behavior with a high propensity to metastasize.

Polymorphous low-grade adenocarcinoma

PLGA occurs almost exclusively in the MiSGs, especially in the palate, buccal mucosa, and upper lip. Cervical metastasis is extremely uncommon in PLGA, except for in the case of cribriform adenocarcinoma of the minor salivary gland (CASMG), which has a greater than 50% incidence of metastases.[21,22]

PREDICTORS OF LYMPH NODE METASTASES

In addition to the subtypes, certain pathologic features are related to higher risk of occult metastases (**Table 1**). These metastases include tumors that are primarily located in the oral cavity, particularly the tongue, or nasopharynx. Similarly, high-grade tumors, especially MEC or salivary ductal, large T3 or T4 tumors, tumors with extraparotid extension, tumors with perilymphatic invasion, or elderly patients presenting with facial paralysis all tend to present with occult cervical metastases. Therefore, these features, or high-grade MEC, AdCC with high-grade degeneration (**Fig. 3**), or salivary ductal, should alert the clinician to perform END.

EVIDENCE FOR LEVEL OF METASTASES AND EXTENT OF DISSECTION

Recommendations for which levels to dissect vary based on T stage and histologic subtype (see **Table 1**). High-risk tumors, including high-grade tumors, large tumors,

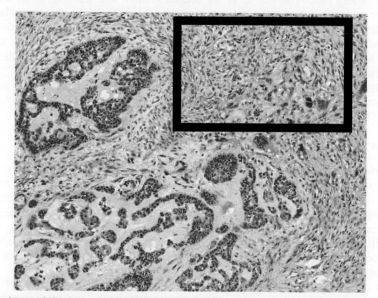

Fig. 3. AdCC with high-grade transformation (dedifferentiation): virtually any salivary gland carcinoma may undergo high-grade transformation. The tumor in the rectangle shows sarcomatoid dedifferentiation (H&E stain; x400).

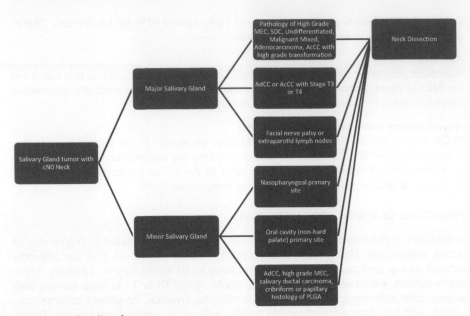

Fig. 4. END, deciding factors.

and special cases like pathologically aggressive, like cribriform adenocarcinoma of MiSG CASMG, and SDC (Salivary Ductal Carcinoma), should be treated with END. With regard to which levels should be dissected, several groups recommend including *at least* levels II to III for major salivary gland disease, I to III for oral cavity as well, whereas others recommend I to III for submandibular and sublingual glands with extension to level IV based on risk assessment.[1,5,17,26–29] Given the potential sites at risk as well as the risk of skip metastases, lymphadenectomy should include levels I to III except for in high-grade MEC and salivary ductal carcinoma (SDC) of the parotid, in which level IV should be included and in those with high-grade MEC and cN+ disease, level V should also be included.[30]

Lymphadenectomy for minor SGC should include levels I to III if within the oral cavity (extrapalatal). For nasopharyngeal carcinoma and high grade parotid carcinoma, level V should be considered if cN+.

SUMMARY

Although ultimately there remains nuance to the decision regarding END for cN0, there are clear indications even given the limited literature (**Fig. 4**). For patients who are poor surgical candidates, radiation can be considered but is not addressed in depth here. For cases whereby the recommendations are unclear, patient comorbidities, pathologic factors, and tumor board recommendations should be considered. Future work with full analysis of the available National Cancer Database to look at the historic rate of occult metastases and prospective work collecting data on cervical lymph node positivity is necessary and underway.

When choosing levels of dissection, lymph node drainage patterns and historical data are useful. Future work with lymphoscintigraphy and intraoperative ultrasound may also be useful in future, prospective assessment of at-risk nodal basins.

CLINICS CARE POINTS

- Elective neck dissection for major salivary gland carcinoma is recommended for the following:
  - High-grade pathologic condition
    - High-grade mucoepidermoid carcinoma and adenoid cystic carcinoma
    - Salivary ductal carcinoma
    - Malignant mixed
    - Adenocarcinoma
  - T3/T4 adenoid cystic carcinoma and acinic cell carcinoma
  - Facial nerve paralysis or perineural spread
  - Periparotid lymph nodes (for example, preauricular lymph nodes or intraparotid lymph nodes)
  - Perilymphatic invasion
  - Extraparenchymal extension
- Elective neck dissection for minor salivary gland carcinoma is recommended for the following:
  - Nasopharyngeal or oral cavity (extrapalatal, hard palate) subsites
  - Pathologic condition
    - Adenoid cystic carcinoma
    - Adenocarcinoma
    - High-grade mucoepidermoid carcinoma
    - Salivary ductal carcinoma
    - Cribriform or papillary histology of polymorphous low-grade adenocarcinoma
- Neck dissection extent:
  - Levels I to V
    - Nasopharyngeal minor salivary gland carcinoma
  - Levels I to IV
    - High-grade mucoepidermoid carcinoma
    - Salivary ductal carcinoma
  - Levels I to III
    - Adenoid cystic carcinoma and acinic cell carcinoma with risk features (see above)
    - Polymorphous low-grade adenocarcinoma with cribriform or papillary histology

ACKNOWLEDGMENTS

Special thanks to Julie Dueber, MD, University of Kentucky and Thèrése Bocklage, MD, University of Kentucky microscopy credit.

DISCLOSURES

Dr A.E. Kejner would like to disclose that she has a completed research grant from Vioptix, Inc.

REFERENCES

1. Byrd S, Morris LGT. Neck dissection for salivary gland malignancies. Oper Tech Otolayngol Head Neck Surg 2018;29(3):157–61.
2. Del Signore AG, Megwalu UC. The rising incidence of major salivary gland cancer in the United States. Ear Nose Throat J 2017;96(3):E13–6.
3. Westergaard-Nielsen M, Rosenberg T, Gerke O, et al. Elective neck dissection in patients with salivary gland carcinoma: a systematic review and meta-analysis. J Oral Pathol Med 2020;49(7):606–16.

4. National comprehensive cancer network. Bone cancer (version 2.2019). Available at: http://www.nccn.org/professionals/physician_gls/pdf/bone.pdf. Accessed April 10.
5. Lau VH, Aouad R, Farwell DG, et al. Patterns of nodal involvement for clinically N0 salivary gland carcinoma: refining the role of elective neck irradiation. Head Neck 2014;36(10):1435–9.
6. Pinkston JA, Cole P. Incidence rates of salivary gland tumors: results from a population-based study. Otolaryngol Head Neck Surg 1999;120(6):834–40.
7. Stenner M, Klussmann JP. Current update on established and novel biomarkers in salivary gland carcinoma pathology and the molecular pathways involved. Eur Arch Otorhinolaryngol 2009;266(3):333–41.
8. Luksic IVM, Manijlovic S. Salivary gland tumors: 25 years of experience from a single institution in Croatia. J Craniomaxillofac Surg 2011;40(3):75–81.
9. Tian Z, Li L, Wang L, et al. Salivary gland neoplasms in oral and maxillofacial regions: a 23-year retrospective study of 6982 cases in an eastern Chinese population. Int J Oral Maxillofac Surg 2010;39(3):235–42.
10. Boukheris H, Curtis RE, Land CE, et al. Incidence of carcinoma of the major salivary glands according to the WHO classification, 1992 to 2006: a population-based study in the United States. Cancer Epidemiol Biomarkers Prev 2009; 18(11):2899–906.
11. Copelli C, Bianchi B, Ferrari S, et al. Malignant tumors of intraoral minor salivary glands. Oral Oncol 2008;44(7):658–63.
12. Mucke T, Robitzky LK, Kesting MR, et al. Advanced malignant minor salivary glands tumors of the oral cavity. Oral Surg Oral Med Oral Pathol Oral Radiol Endod 2009;108(1):81–9.
13. Karatayli-Ozgursoy SBJ, Hillel AT, Akst LM, et al. Malignant salivary gland tumours of the larynx: a single institution review. Tumori maligni delle ghiandole salivari della laringe: un'unica review istituzionale. Acta Otorhinolaryngol Ital 2016; 36(4):289–94.
14. Ellington CL, Goodman M, Kono SA, et al. Adenoid cystic carcinoma of the head and neck: incidence and survival trends based on 1973-2007 Surveillance, Epidemiology, and End Results data. Cancer 2012;118(18):4444–51.
15. Lee A, Givi B, Osborn VW, et al. Patterns of care and survival of adjuvant radiation for major salivary adenoid cystic carcinoma. Laryngoscope 2017;127(9): 2057–62.
16. Ko JJ, Siever JE, Hao D, et al. Adenoid cystic carcinoma of head and neck: clinical predictors of outcome from a Canadian centre. Curr Oncol 2016;23(1):26–33.
17. Armstrong JG, Harrison LB, Thaler HT, et al. The indications for elective treatment of the neck in cancer of the major salivary glands. Cancer 1992;69(3):615–9.
18. Sood S, Mcgurk M, Vaz F. Management of salivary gland tumours: United Kingdom National Multidisciplinary Guidelines. J Laryngol Otol 2016;130(Suppl. S2):S142–9.
19. Grasl S, Janik S, Grasl MC, et al. Nodal metastases in acinic cell carcinoma of the parotid gland. J Clin Med 2019;8(9):1315.
20. Fang Q, Wu J, Du W, et al. Predictors of distant metastasis in parotid acinic cell carcinoma. BMC Cancer 2019;19(1):475.
21. Michal M, Kacerovska D, Kazakov DV. Cribriform adenocarcinoma of the tongue and minor salivary glands: a review. Head Neck Pathol 2013;7(Suppl 1):S3–11.
22. Skalova A, Sima R, Kaspirkova-Nemcova J, et al. Cribriform adenocarcinoma of minor salivary gland origin principally affecting the tongue: characterization of new entity. Am J Surg Pathol 2011;35(8):1168–76.

23. Chen MM, Roman SA, Sosa JA, et al. Histologic grade as prognostic indicator for mucoepidermoid carcinoma: a population-level analysis of 2400 patients. Head Neck 2014;36(2):158–63.
24. Xiao CC, Zhan KY, White-Gilbertson SJ, et al. Predictors of nodal metastasis in parotid malignancies: a National Cancer Data Base study of 22,653 patients. Otolaryngol Head Neck Surg 2016;154(1):121–30.
25. International H, Neck Scientific G. Cervical lymph node metastasis in adenoid cystic carcinoma of the major salivary glands. J Laryngol Otol 2017;131(2): 96–105.
26. Mantravadi AVMM, Rassekh CH. AHNS series: do you know your guidelines? Diagnosis and management of salivary gland tumors. Head Neck 2019;41(2): 269–80.
27. Wang XLY, Li M, Yan H, et al. Management of salivary gland carcinomas - a review. Oncotarget 2017;8(3):3946–56.
28. Som PMB-GM. Anatomy and pathology of the salivary glands. In: Som PMCH, editor. Head and neck imaging. 5th edition. St. Louis (MO): Mosby; 2011. p. 2449–602.
29. Grossman RIYD. Extramucosal diseases of the head and neck. In: Grossman RIYD, editor. Neuroradiology: the requisites. 3rd edition. St. Louis (MO): Mosby; 2010. p. 476–514.
30. Lim CM, Gilbert M, Johnson JT, et al. Is level V neck dissection necessary in primary parotid cancer? Laryngoscope 2015;125(1):118–21.

Special Article Series: Intentionally Shaping the Future of Otolaryngology

Editor

JENNIFER A. VILLWOCK

OTOLARYNGOLOGIC CLINICS OF NORTH AMERICA

www.oto.theclinics.com

Consulting Editor
SUJANA S. CHANDRASEKHAR

June 2021 • Volume 54 • Number 3

Foreword
Turning Dreams and Goals into Plans and Actions that Enhance Otolaryngology

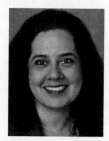

Sujana S. Chandrasekhar, MD, FACS, FAAOHNS
Consulting Editor

Antoine de Saint-Exupéry, poet and author of *The Little Prince*, hero fighter pilot who perished in World War II, famously said, "A goal without a plan is just a wish." Extrapolating from that, a goal with a plan becomes an action. A well-thought-out plan that uses data effectively allows that action to achieve the goal.

Thus far, the articles in the Special Article Series: Intentionally Shaping the Future of Otolaryngology in prior issues of *Otolaryngologic Clinics of North America* have established the data regarding our specialty in terrific detail. As Guest Editor, Dr Jennifer Villwock spearheads this series of articles, which appear two at a time. The first articles were on Leadership and the dearth of diversity therein and appeared in the August 2020 issue. The articles in the October 2020 issue covered the current state of the Otolaryngology workforce and defined diversity among our peers and why it is important. The February 2021 articles discussed the challenging history of women and minorities in surgery and took a deep dive into leadership competencies in medicine. In April 2021, we learned about mentorship and sponsorship in a diverse population and about diversity in Otolaryngologic training.

The 2 articles in the current issue offer concrete and actionable ideas for diversifying research and funding and outline critical components when establishing diversity initiatives. This work is difficult but important, if we are to shape our field to truly represent our physicians and allied health personnel, and the patients whom we serve.

A prime example is Research Project Grant (R01) funding from the National Institutes of Health (NIH). The R01 is the original and historically oldest grant mechanism used by NIH. It provides support for health-related research and development.[1] An R01 is a mature award that gives the investigator 4 or 5 years of independent support, enough money and time to complete a project, publish results, and start writing their next

Otolaryngol Clin N Am 54 (2021) xvii–xix
https://doi.org/10.1016/j.otc.2021.04.009
0030-6665/21/© 2021 Published by Elsevier Inc.

application in time to get an award before the funding ends. A study[2] looked at 6 minority medical schools compared with 6 nonminority medical schools. In the minority medical schools, only 15% ± 4% of the total NIH support went to R01-type funding, whereas 65% ± 11% of the total NIH support went to R01-type funding at nonminority institutions. Dr J. Anderson Eloy's article on Diversifying Research and Funding explores this pipeline problem in detail and provides methods for ameliorating it.

DEI seems to be the current buzz term. It stands for Diversity, Equity, and Inclusion, and institutions are scrambling to fill leadership positions in their nascent diversity initiatives. The article by Drs Brandon Ithiel Esianor, Cristina Cabrera-Muffly, Nicole Kloosterman, David Brown, and Kimberly Vinson on Critical Components of Diversity Initiatives explores how a successful DEI initiative goes from being a token entry on a Web site to being a meaningful part of that institution. This requires being embedded in the institution's Leadership, Human Resources, and Strategic Planning, with adequate authority and resources so that timely and measurable progress toward clearly defined milestones becomes the fabric of the entire institution.

Once again, I thank Dr Villwock for editing this exceptional Special Series, from which we all benefit. Each article provides much needed food for thought. Please take the time to read them and share them with your teams.

Sujana S. Chandrasekhar, MD, FACS, FAAOHNS
Consulting Editor
Otolaryngologic Clinics of North America
Past President
American Academy of Otolaryngology–
Head and Neck Surgery
Secretary-Treasurer
American Otological Society
Partner, ENT & Allergy Associates LLP
18 East 48th Street, 2nd Floor
New York, NY 10017, USA

Clinical Professor, Department of Otolaryngology–
Head and Neck Surgery
Zucker School of Medicine at Hofstra-Northwell
Hempstead, NY, USA

Clinical Associate Professor
Department of Otolaryngology–
Head and Neck Surgery
Icahn School of Medicine at Mount Sinai
New York, NY, USA

E-mail address:
ssc@nyotology.com

Website:
http://www.ears.nyc

REFERENCES

1. Available at: https://grants.nih.gov/grants/funding/r01.htm#:~:text=Introduction, via%20a%20Request%20for%20Applications. Accessed March 27, 2021.
2. Guers JJ, Gwathmey J, Haddad G, et al. A potential solution to the continuing problem of not enough NIH R01 funding to minority investigators. FASEB J 2017;31:750.11. https://doi.org/10.1096/fasebj.31.1_supplement.750.11. Available at:.

Preface
From Desire to Doing

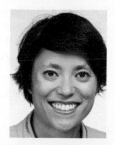

Jennifer A. Villwock, MD
Editor

Most who are called to medicine have a deeply rooted desire to make a positive impact on their patients and their communities. There are numerous ways to do this, ranging from clinical care, community service, research, teaching, outreach, and so on. However, one thing is constant in these pursuits. It is not enough to simply *want* to have this impact. The appropriate actions and actually doing the work are required. It goes without saying that to be a physician, medical school is required. To become a board-certified otolaryngologist, completion of 5 years of residency and successful passage of written and oral board exams must occur. Without the work, the dream cannot become a reality.

The same is true for pursuing the goals of equity, diversity, and justice within our field and society. Desire alone is insufficient. We must also do.

In their article "Diversifying Research and Funding," Dr Eloy and colleagues provide compelling evidence regarding disparities in research funding that impacts the longitudinal trajectory of otolaryngologists and the research questions our field explores.

Dr Esianor's team then provides concrete recommendations that build upon this knowledge base in their piece, "Critical Components of Diversity Initiatives." We are accustomed to seeing and answering the following question about clinical scenarios: What is the next most appropriate step in management? Dr Esianor and colleagues provide answers to this question in the context of building and sustaining meaningful diversity, equity, and inclusion initiatives that can be used in any setting.

Otolaryngol Clin N Am 54 (2021) xxi–xxii
https://doi.org/10.1016/j.otc.2021.03.003
0030-6665/21/© 2021 Published by Elsevier Inc.

oto.theclinics.com

It is our hope that these special articles add to the reader's repertoire of knowledge and skills to better transition from desiring equity, diversity, and justice to taking discrete actions to bring this dream to fruition.

Jennifer A. Villwock, MD
Department of Otolaryngology
Head and Neck Surgery
University of Kansas Medical Center
3901 Rainbow Boulevard, MS 3010
Kansas City, KS 66160, USA

E-mail address:
jvillwock@kumc.edu

Diversifying Researchers and Funding in Otolaryngology

Christina H. Fang, MD[a], Gregory L. Barinsky, PharmD[a],
Stacey T. Gray, MD[b,c], Soly Baredes, MD[a,d],
Sujana S. Chandrasekhar, MD[e], Jean Anderson Eloy, MD[a,d,f,g,h,*]

KEYWORDS

- Diversity • Equity • Otolaryngology • Gender • Racial • Ethnicity • Research
- Grant funding

KEY POINTS

- Gender disparity exists in academic Otolaryngology, specifically in scholarly productivity, representation at national conferences, leadership of journal editorial boards, and grant funding.
- Ethnic and racial disparities in Otolaryngology grant funding have been identified.
- Disparity in academic advancement in Otolaryngology may be precipitated by these inequalities in scholarly performance.
- Actionable measures for diverse trainee and faculty recruitment, retention, and promotion are necessary to reach equity in Otolaryngology.

Financial Disclosures: None.
[a] Department of Otolaryngology – Head and Neck Surgery, Rutgers New Jersey Medical School, Newark, NJ, USA; [b] Department of Otolaryngology – Head and Neck Surgery, Harvard Medical School, Boston, MA, USA; [c] Department of Otolaryngology – Head and Neck Surgery, Massachusetts Eye and Ear, Boston, MA, USA; [d] Center for Skull Base and Pituitary Surgery, Neurological Institute of New Jersey, Rutgers New Jersey Medical School, Newark, NJ, USA; [e] ENT & Allergy Associates, LLP, Zucker School of Medicine at Hofstra-Northwell, Icahn School of Medicine at Mount Sinai, New York, NY, USA; [f] Department of Neurological Surgery, Rutgers New Jersey Medical School, Newark, NJ, USA; [g] Department of Ophthalmology and Visual Science, Rutgers New Jersey Medical School, Newark, NJ, USA; [h] Department of Otolaryngology and Facial Plastic Surgery, Saint Barnabas Medical Center - RWJBarnabas Health, Livingston, NJ, USA
* Corresponding author. Rhinology and Sinus Surgery, Otolaryngology Research, Endoscopic Skull Base Surgery Program, Department of Otolaryngology – Head and Neck Surgery, Neurological Institute of New Jersey, Rutgers New Jersey Medical School, 90 Bergen Street, Suite 8100, Newark, NJ 07103.
E-mail address: jean.anderson.eloy@gmail.com

INTRODUCTION

Academic rank and leadership positions are measures of career progression in academic medicine. Research productivity metrics play an integral role in professional development, because advancement and promotion are heavily based on publications and grant funding. There are known gender, race, and ethnicity disparities in Otolaryngology, specifically with regards to research and grant funding. This article discusses these disparities, the professional implications, and the approaches by which the specialty can make concerted efforts to promote equity.

GENDER DISPARITY IN OTOLARYNGOLOGY RESEARCH PRODUCTIVITY

A stark gender disparity exists in Otolaryngology. The proportion of women medical students has been rising recently, from 46.9% in 2015 to 49.5% in 2018 to 50.5% in 2019. However, as of 2018, women made up 35.6% of the 1542 otolaryngology resident physicians in the United States (US).[1] Furthermore, women comprise a low percentage of academic otolaryngologists (34.6% in 2019) and are further underrepresented in leadership positions.[2] In 2019, women comprised 37.8% of assistant professors, 28.3% of associate professors, and 16.0% of professors.[3] In 2018, of 86 US academic otolaryngology departments, three had female chairs.[4] Several factors have been postulated to account for this gender disparity, including lack of female role models, directing a greater proportion of professional effort to teaching and patient care compared with research, work-life balance concerns, and conscious or unconscious gender bias and discrimination.[5-10] As a result, there are fewer women in academic positions available to provide gender-concordant mentoring for junior female colleagues.[11,12]

Academic otolaryngologists are evaluated for promotion based on their clinical productivity, research contributions, and administrative and educational roles. Academic productivity is often assessed by the number and significance of publications, citations, research grants, and other accolades.[13,14] The h-index, first described by Hirsch[14] in 2005, provides a measure of the number (h) of articles published that have a minimum of h citations each. This metric takes into account the significance of the published work and provides a measure of quality and impact.[15] The h-index is used as a surrogate for scholarly productivity in the literature, with higher values associated with increased research productivity, promotion, and academic rank.[16,17]

Female academic otolaryngologists have been shown to have lower academic productivity during the early years of their careers. Eloy and colleagues[7] found that female assistant and associate professors have significantly lower h-indices when compared with their male counterparts. In contrast, female professors and chairs had higher h-indices than males of the same rank, although this was not statistically significant. They did find, however, that the difference in h-indices between male and female academic otolaryngologists disappeared after 20 years of research experience. This suggests that women later in their career, have more time to dedicate to academic and research productivity. Thus, early career considerations unique to female otolaryngologists may need to be taken into account when evaluating for promotion.[18] Another possibility for this difference is that historically and more so today, men self-cite their own work in their publications 56% more than do women, in a study of 1.5 million papers between 1779 and 2011.[19] Although many of these citations may be appropriate, these may drive the h-index up in a potentially artificial manner. Moreover, one cannot cite themselves for work that one was not permitted or encouraged to do. A follow-up study of this gender gap was conducted in 2019 using the e-index, which is comprised of all publications of an individual that have a certain number (h) of citations.[20] The e-index is a useful complement to the h-index that addresses some of its limitations.[20] Overall, male academic otolaryngologists continued to have higher research productivity, measured by the h-index, e-index, number of citations, and active publishing years.[21] Encouragingly, however, women seemed to be keeping pace with their male counterparts in the early career period (<15 years) in certain subfields of Otolaryngology. This represents a change from previous findings,[7] and is potentially secondary to evolving gender roles in home and childcare responsibilities and women postponing pregnancy until later in their careers.[21] In addition, this may be caused by increased awareness of the current gender gap in scholarly productivity and perhaps increased encouragement of female residents and fellows to pursue research and funding.

GENDER DISPARITY IN SCHOLARLY PRODUCTIVITY IN OTHER SPECIALTIES

Gender disparity in research productivity is not unique to Otolaryngology. In specialty-specific studies, female academic plastic surgeons, ophthalmologists, gynecologic oncologists, and anesthesiologists have been shown to have significantly lower early career research productivity when compared with males.[22–25] A review of 9952 US academic physicians in 34 different medical specialties similarly found that female faculty members have lower research productivity when stratified by rank.[26] In academic neurosurgery, women overall had lower scholarly productivity, but this difference disappeared when comparing productivity within cohorts of similar academic rank.[27]

FEMALE AUTHORSHIP AND JOURNAL LEADERSHIP IN OTOLARYNGOLOGY

A study examining journal authorship in Otolaryngology suggests that women are producing proportionate academic output. Bergeron and colleagues[28] found that the proportion of female authorship in Otolaryngology journals has significantly increased from 14.5% to 22.5% between 1978 and 2008. A significant proportion of the female authors (19.2%), however, were nonphysicians. The prevalence of female first authorship was found to be 21.3%. Of note, this is greater than the proportion of actively practicing female Otolaryngologists in the US of approximately 11% in 2008.[29]

A study of authorship of scientific opinion articles in leading Otolaryngology journals between 2013 and 2018 found that the proportion of female first authorship increased from 20.0% to 32.0%.[30] In addition, the proportion of women among physician first authors (27.1%) was significantly greater than the percentage of actively practicing female otolaryngologists (17.1%). Female first authors were more likely than male first authors to have female last authors, which suggests mentorship and collaboration among women in Otolaryngology.

Litvack and colleagues[31] examined the presence of women on the editorial boards of nine clinical otolaryngology journals. They found that female board membership increased from 7.2% to 17.7% over a 20-year period (1997–2017). However, this proportion remained significantly less than the proportion of female US otolaryngology faculty of 28% in 2017. In addition, none of these journals had a female editor-in-chief during this time period. It seems that although female authorship in Otolaryngology has risen proportionally, leadership roles in publishing remain heavily dominated by men.

GENDER REPRESENTATION AT OTOLARYNGOLOGY CONFERENCES

Presentation of research and involvement in scientific panels at academic conferences are linked to career advancement. Meeting participation creates networking opportunities and enhances visibility and name recognition. Barinsky and colleagues[32] examined gender representation among speakers, oral session moderators, panelists, executive board members, program committee members, and citation recipients at three national otolaryngology conferences. From 2005 to 2018, there has been an increase in the proportion of women occupying these opportunity spots, growing from 16.9% to 29.5%. In addition, the number of male-only panels decreased from 87.5% to 24.0% over the same time period. Further analysis showed, however, that on average' there was one unique woman for every four opportunity spots filled by women, suggesting that the same women account for a large proportion of increased female representation at these meetings. It is possible that women may have less national and international recognition, a factor commonly used when inviting speakers and panelists to conferences,[33] but because junior men are frequently mentored into one or several of these opportunity spots, this could be a function of either conscious or unconscious bias.

GENDER IN OTOLARYNGOLOGY RESEARCH FUNDING

Identifying and retaining academic faculty with the ability to secure grants and external funding for research is advantageous for all institutions. As the leading governmental supporter of funding for biomedical research in the US the National Institutes of Health (NIH) provides the ideal benchmark for us to study. Research (R) grants are the most common funding mechanisms by which the NIH supports investigators at all levels.

Gender disparity among NIH awards for otolaryngology faculty has been identified.[18,34] Male otolaryngology faculty were found to have higher overall NIH funding (mean, $498,593 \pm $43,407) compared with their female counterparts (mean, $359,276 \pm $64,406).[18] When controlling for academic rank, the difference in NIH funding was found to be significant beginning at the level of assistant professor, where both genders were nearly equally represented. Significant differences were also found when comparing male and female faculty with 10 to 20 years of experience. In addition, the most coveted R-Series research grants were awarded in greater proportion to men, and those awarded to male investigators were for greater amounts than those awarded to women. Unsurprisingly, scholarly impact has also been shown to be associated with greater NIH awards among academic otolaryngologists.[35] Hence, a gender gap in obtaining research funding may contribute to the disparity in research productivity. Similar to previously discussed findings, these data suggest that early career female faculty may be at a disadvantage.

An alternate source for research funding, especially for early career otolaryngologists, includes grants from the Centralized Otolaryngology Research Efforts (CORE) program. Created in 1985, the CORE program is a collaboration between several otolaryngology societies, foundations, and industry supporters that provides support for research projects, training, and career development.[36] There is a strong correlation between CORE grant funding and scholarly achievement, with CORE grant-funded academic otolaryngologists having significantly higher h-indices than their non-CORE grant-funded academic peers.[37] Procurement of a CORE grant has also been associated with future receipt of NIH funding.[38]

Analysis of 310 CORE grant recipients over a 10-year period (2010–2019) found that the proportion of female grant recipients remained nearly unchanged (39.1%–40.0%) (Roy and colleagues, unpublished data, September 2020). When comparing this with the proportion of female otolaryngology residents (35.6% in 2018) and female faculty members in the United States (34.6% in 2019), there seems to be a small but relative outperformance of women in obtaining CORE grants.[1,2] Given that CORE grant funding is positively correlated with likelihood of NIH funding and overall research productivity, this may be a promising finding. It is hoped that the downstream effects of highly productive early career female otolaryngologists in recent years will narrow the current gender gap.

GENDER AND INDUSTRY FUNDING IN OTOLARYNGOLOGY

Collaboration with the medical industry has the potential to promote scholarly discourse and increase accessibility to novel technology and therapeutics. In 2010, the Open Payments Program of the Centers for Medicare and Medicaid Services introduced mandatory public reporting of payments made to physicians by medical device and pharmaceutical companies.[39] Established by the Physician Payments Sunshine Act, this database increases the transparency of physician-industry relationships.

The impact of gender on industry support in academic otolaryngology has been previously evaluated using Open Payments data. In 2014, of 992 academic otolaryngologists with industry relationships, men received higher contributions (median, $211; interquartile range, $86–$1245) than women (median, $133; interquartile range, $51–$316).[40] This difference held true when controlling for academic rank, specifically at the assistant and associate professor level. In addition, a greater proportion of men received contributions from industry than women (68.0% vs 56.1%). Similar gender-based differences in industry payments have also been shown to exist in academic neurosurgery.[41,42]

Industry inherently values academic productivity, because it demonstrates expertise and establishes an individual as a key opinion and thought leader. Otolaryngologists who receive industry support for research purposes have significantly greater scholarly productivity, as measured by the h-index.[43] By partnering with prominent otolaryngologists, companies are able to lend credibility to their device or medication. Because female otolaryngologists do not publish as much as males early on in their careers, they may not be identified by companies as a desirable collaborator. This potentially extends the time in practice necessary to establish a strong industry relationship. Data also suggest the possibility of an inherent bias, because academic merit (ie, publications) is a greater determinant of industry payment to women than to men.[42]

Industry funding seems to be closely intertwined with academic advancement: productivity is aided by funding, productivity drives academic ranking, and ranking drives funding.[44] Thus, if gender inequality in industry funding is a downstream effect of disparities in metrics of productivity, these areas must first be addressed before funding parity can be achieved.

ETHNIC AND RACIAL DISPARITY IN OTOLARYNGOLOGY RESEARCH

In 2014, the Association of American Medical Colleges defined "underrepresented in medicine" as those racial and ethnic populations underrepresented in the medical profession relative to their numbers in the general population.[45] This is a change from their prior definition, which only included four racial and ethnic groups: (1) Blacks, (2) Mexican-Americans, (3) Native Americans, and (4) mainland Puerto Ricans. Blacks and Hispanics remain underrepresented in medical school, and even more so in Otolaryngology. Their representation decreases along the academic otolaryngology pipeline as rank increases.[46] As of 2019, the proportion of Black and Hispanic otolaryngology faculty members remains low, at 1.9% and 3.0%, respectively.[2]

To date, there has been little study of racial and ethnic disparities in otolaryngology research productivity and funding. Although underrepresented minorities have been shown to be less successful in obtaining NIH grant funding in general, specific studies in Otolaryngology have yet to be conducted.[47,48] In a review of CORE grant recipients in 2010 and 2019, most grant recipients were White (63.0% and 69.7%, respectively) (Roy and colleagues, unpublished data, September 2020). In 2010, Black and Hispanic recipients made up 2.2% and 2.2% of grant recipients, respectively. In 2019, these numbers were the same or worse: Blacks and Hispanics accounted for 3.0% and 0.0% of grant funding, respectively.

DISPARITY IN OTOLARYNGOLOGY FACULTY RANK

The underrepresentation of women and racial/ethnic minorities in academic medicine is often explained by citing a cohort effect: that an overall shift in faculty demographics naturally occurs in parallel with the increasing number of women and minorities in the general population.[49] However, studies have shown that changes in the diversity of medical faculty do not take place at this expected rate.[17,50]

Because academic productivity is closely tied to promotion, disparity in research productivity and grant funding is likely a major cause of the underrepresentation of female and minority otolaryngologists in academic leadership positions. Men have higher representation at senior academic ranks, a trend that seems to be consistent throughout several geographic regions in the US.[17] In addition, women are underrepresented in leadership positions, such as residency/fellowship directorships, and departmental and division chair positions.[51] This gender disparity among faculty rank in academic departments is not unique to Otolaryngology and is present in almost every field of medicine. Specifically, a review of 11,549 academic surgeons found that women were less likely than men to be professors after adjusting for factors known to impact faculty rank.[10] Encouragingly, however, women have been shown to be taking on directorship roles while having lower academic ranks, less years of practice, and lower h-indices, suggesting a trend toward earlier involvement in leadership.[51]

The decrease in the number of minority physicians along the academic promotion pipeline is more pronounced in Otolaryngology than in other areas of medicine.[46] Underrepresented minorities have been shown to have lower rates of promotion and retention.[52,53] Nonspecific specialty data have also shown that minority physicians are more likely to report considering leaving academia.[54] In addition to racial discrimination and promotion bias, unequal distribution of research time and clinical support have been identified as challenges faced by minority faculty.[50] Underrepresented faculty are often subject to the "minority tax," which are extra responsibilities placed on minority faculty by an institution in the name of efforts to improve diversity.[55,56] For example, they may be asked to take on an institution's community efforts in areas of diversity, which are generally neither recompensed nor as highly regarded in the evaluation for promotion.[57] In addition, academic minority physicians often care for underserved populations in greater numbers than their nonminority colleagues.[58,59] Thus, the increase in clinical and diversity-related demands leaves less time for scholarly and research activities that are vital for promotion.

LIMITATIONS

The studies discussed within this article have several limitations that should be kept in mind. Most studies were retrospective in nature and do not allow for attribution of causality. The h-index was a commonly used surrogate for scholarly productivity, but is not without drawbacks. This metric clearly favors individuals later in their careers, because they have been producing published works for a longer period of time that can be cited by others. Thus, a lower h-index in a younger faculty member does not necessarily indicate poor research productivity.[60] In addition, the h-index may be potentially inflated by self-citation.[61] However, the repeated and sustained self-citation needed to do so would be significant and is likely difficult to accomplish at higher h-indices.

FUTURE DIRECTIONS IN ACHIEVING PARITY

Despite these limitations, there is clear evidence of distinct gender, racial, and ethnic disparities in otolaryngology research and funding. This, in turn, likely contributes to a disparity in academic promotion and advancement among female and minority otolaryngologists. Further studies are necessary to determine the underlying reasons these disparities exist.

The importance of diverse perspectives in otolaryngology research should be stressed, because diversity brings innovative thought and new problem-solving skills to the field. Early exposure to otolaryngology research is pivotal for underrepresented minorities and women, because research and publications are imperative to entering a competitive specialty. Some recommend that otolaryngology departments invite undergraduate and medical students from diverse backgrounds to attend conferences and didactics.[46] In addition, early exposure to committed mentors can encourage underrepresented students to pursue academic careers. At a national level, the Society of University Otolaryngologists supports underrepresented medical students by providing funding for clinical and research rotations.

The need for female leaders in Otolaryngology has been recognized by the American Academy of Otolaryngology – Head and Neck Surgery. The Women in Otolaryngology Section was designed to promote female leadership and mentorship. Specifically, the Women in Otolaryngology Endowment Grants fund projects that seek to explore and advance the success of women in Otolaryngology. With more than 2000 members joining since its inception 10 years ago, support for this initiative is strong and continues to increase.

In academic otolaryngology, aggressive measures for female and minority faculty recruitment, retention, and promotion are necessary to reach parity. Training to minimize implicit bias throughout the recruitment and promotion process should be implemented. Recognizing that minority responsibility and workload disparity exists, institutions should seek to value these efforts with support and recognition. Adjusting assignment of such responsibilities to allow greater research or academic time and ensuring that clinical and community efforts are counted toward promotion can help retain and advance underrepresented faculty.[50] Such interventions will likely be more successful if they acknowledge the unique burdens that underrepresented faculty face.

Given the disparity present in research funding, consideration should be given to blinding applications, specifically to name, gender, and institution. This would allow for the evaluation of proposed grants to be performed without bias. In addition, it is important to mandate greater diversity at academic conferences and on scientific panels because this can improve attendees' experiences and encourage minorities to participate in scientific discourse. Promoting a diverse student, trainee, and faculty population in Otolaryngology will lead to a more robust learning environment for all.[45] As a unified field, we should continue to strive for parity and for understanding and addressing our own implicit biases, and should inequalities be identified, push ourselves to make changes until parity is obtained.

SUMMARY

Gender, racial, and ethnic disparities exist in otolaryngology research productivity and funding. Specifically, women academic otolaryngologists lag in scholarly productivity, representation at national conferences, leadership of journal editorial boards, and grant funding when compared with their male counterparts. In addition, not only were men more likely than women to receive NIH and industry funding, but they also received greater amounts of payment. Studies examining racial and ethnic disparities are lacking in comparison. Blacks and Hispanics have been shown to receive the lowest proportion of CORE grant research funding when compared with nonminority otolaryngologists. Because scholarly productivity is an important factor taken into consideration for promotion, these disparities may account for the disproportionate number of women and underrepresented minorities in higher ranks and leadership positions in academic otolaryngology. With these findings in mind, implementation of directed approaches is necessary to move the specialty toward parity. This includes early research exposure and research funding for women and underrepresented minorities. It is also imperative to understand the role of implicit bias and the impact of the "minority tax" when evaluating women and minorities during the academic recruitment and promotion process.

CLINICS CARE POINTS

- It is important to acknowledge and address the racial disparities in academic otolaryngology with regards to research productivity and grant funding.
- Awareness of these disparities and directed approaches aid in recruiting and retaining diverse otolaryngology faculty.
- Early exposure to otolaryngology research is pivotal for underrepresented minorities and women, because research and publications are important for academic advancement.
- Training to minimize implicit bias and recognition of the minority workload disparity should be implemented by academic institutions.

CONFLICTS OF INTEREST

None.

REFERENCES

1. Colleges AoAM. Number of active residents by type of medical school, GME specialty, and sex. Available at: https://www.aamc.org/data-reports/students-residents/interactive-data/table-b3-number-active-residents-type-medical-school-gme-specialty-and-sex. Accessed September 9, 2020.
2. Colleges AoAM. Table 16: US medical school faculty by sex, race/ethnicity, and department. 2019. Available at: https://www.aamc.org/system/files/2020-01/2019Table16.pdf. Accessed September 16, 2020.
3. Colleges AoAM. US medical school faculty by sex, rank, and department. 2019. Available at: https://www.aamc.org/system/files/2020-01/2019Table13.pdf. Accessed September 9, 2020.
4. Colleges AoAM. Department chairs by gender and department. 2018. Available at: https://www.aamc.org/sites/default/files/aa-data-reports-state-of-women-department-chairs-2018_0.jpg. Accessed September 9, 2020.
5. Kuehn BM. More women choose careers in surgery: bias, work-life issues remain challenges. JAMA 2012;307:1899–901.
6. Sanfey HA, Saalwachter-Schulman AR, Nyhof-Young JM, et al. Influences on medical student career choice: gender or generation? Arch Surg 2006;141: 1086–94 [discussion: 1094].

7. Eloy JA, Svider P, Chandrasekhar SS, et al. Gender disparities in scholarly productivity within academic otolaryngology departments. Otolaryngol Head Neck Surg 2013;148:215–22.

8. Reed DA, Enders F, Lindor R, et al. Gender differences in academic productivity and leadership appointments of physicians throughout academic careers. Acad Med 2011;86:43–7.

9. Shea S, Nickerson KG, Tenenbaum J, et al. Compensation to a department of medicine and its faculty members for the teaching of medical students and house staff. N Engl J Med 1996;334:162–7.

10. Blumenthal DM, Bergmark RW, Raol N, et al. Sex differences in faculty rank among academic surgeons in the United States in 2014. Ann Surg 2018;268:193–200.

11. Mayer AP, Files JA, Ko MG, et al. Academic advancement of women in medicine: do socialized gender differences have a role in mentoring? Mayo Clin Proc 2008;83:204–7.

12. Levinson W, Kaufman K, Clark B, et al. Mentors and role models for women in academic medicine. West J Med 1991;154:423–6.

13. von Bohlen Und Halbach O. How to judge a book by its cover? How useful are bibliometric indices for the evaluation of "scientific quality" or "scientific productivity"? Ann Anat 2011;193:191–6.

14. Hirsch JE. An index to quantify an individual's scientific research output. Proc Natl Acad Sci U S A 2005;102:16569–72.

15. Gaster N, Gaster M. A critical assessment of the h-index. Bioessays 2012;34:830–2.

16. Svider PF, Choudhry ZA, Choudhry OJ, et al. The use of the h-index in academic otolaryngology. Laryngoscope 2013;123:103–6.

17. Eloy JA, Mady LJ, Svider PF, et al. Regional differences in gender promotion and scholarly productivity in otolaryngology. Otolaryngol Head Neck Surg 2014;150:371–7.

18. Eloy JA, Svider PF, Kovalerchik O, et al. Gender differences in successful NIH grant funding in otolaryngology. Otolaryngol Head Neck Surg 2013;149:77–83.

19. King MM, Bergstrom CT, Correll SJ, et al. Men set their own cites high: gender and self-citation across fields and over time. Socius: Sociological Research for a Dynamic World 2017;3:1–22.

20. Zhang CT. The e-index, complementing the h-index for excess citations. PLoS One 2009;4:e5429.

21. Okafor S, Tibbetts K, Shah G, et al. Is the gender gap closing in otolaryngology subspecialties? An analysis of research productivity. Laryngoscope 2020;130:1144–50.

22. Paik AM, Mady LJ, Villanueva NL, et al. Research productivity and gender disparities: a look at academic plastic surgery. J Surg Educ 2014;71:593–600.

23. Lopez SA, Svider PF, Misra P, et al. Gender differences in promotion and scholarly impact: an analysis of 1400 academic ophthalmologists. J Surg Educ 2014;71:851–9.

24. Hill EK, Blake RA, Emerson JB, et al. Gender differences in scholarly productivity within academic gynecologic oncology departments. Obstet Gynecol 2015;126:1279–84.

25. Pashkova AA, Svider PF, Chang CY, et al. Gender disparity among US anaesthesiologists: are women underrepresented in academic ranks and scholarly productivity? Acta Anaesthesiol Scand 2013;57:1058–64.

26. Eloy JA, Svider PF, Cherla DV, et al. Gender disparities in research productivity among 9952 academic physicians. Laryngoscope 2013;123:1865–75.
27. Tomei KL, Nahass MM, Husain Q, et al. A gender-based comparison of academic rank and scholarly productivity in academic neurological surgery. J Clin Neurosci 2014;21:1102–5.
28. Bergeron JL, Wilken R, Miller ME, et al. Measurable progress in female authorship in otolaryngology. Otolaryngol Head Neck Surg 2012;147:40–3.
29. Colleges AoAM. Physician specialty data. 2008. Available at: https://www.aamc.org/system/files/reports/1/specialtydata.pdf. Accessed September 9, 2020.
30. Miller AL, Rathi VK, Gray ST, et al. Female authorship of opinion pieces in leading otolaryngology journals between 2013 and 2018. Otolaryngol Head Neck Surg 2020;162:35–7.
31. Litvack JR, Wick EH, Whipple ME. Trends in female leadership at high-profile otolaryngology journals, 1997-2017. Laryngoscope 2019;129:2031–5.
32. Barinsky GL, Daoud D, Tan D, et al. Gender representation at conferences, executive boards, and program committees in otolaryngology. Laryngoscope 2021; 131(2):E373–9.
33. Jagsi R, Guancial EA, Worobey CC, et al. The "gender gap" in authorship of academic medical literature: a 35-year perspective. N Engl J Med 2006;355:281–7.
34. Lennon CJ, Hunter JB, Mistry AM, et al. NIH funding within otolaryngology: 2005-2014. Otolaryngol Head Neck Surg 2017;157:774–80.
35. Svider PF, Mauro KM, Sanghvi S, et al. Is NIH funding predictive of greater research productivity and impact among academic otolaryngologists? Laryngoscope 2013;123:118–22.
36. Surgery AAoO-HaN. CORE grants. Available at: https://www.entnet.org/content/centralized-otolaryngology-research-efforts-core-grants-program. Accessed September 16, 2020.
37. Eloy JA, Svider PF, Folbe AJ, et al. AAO-HNSF CORE grant acquisition is associated with greater scholarly impact. Otolaryngol Head Neck Surg 2014;150:53–60.
38. Eloy JA, Svider PF, Kanumuri VV, et al. Do AAO-HNSF CORE grants predicT FUTUre NIH funding success? Otolaryngol Head Neck Surg 2014;151:246–52.
39. Agrawal S, Brennan N, Budetti P. The sunshine act: effects on physicians. N Engl J Med 2013;368:2054–7.
40. Eloy JA, Bobian M, Svider PF, et al. Association of gender with financial relationships between industry and academic otolaryngologists. JAMA Otolaryngol Head Neck Surg 2017;143:796–802.
41. Eloy JA, Kilic S, Yoo NG, et al. Is industry funding associated with greater scholarly impact among academic neurosurgeons? World Neurosurg 2017;103: 517–25.
42. Ngaage LM, Harris C, Gao C, et al. Investigating the gender pay gap in industry contributions to academic neurosurgeons. World Neurosurg 2019;130: 516–22.e1.
43. Svider PF, Bobian M, Lin HS, et al. Are industry financial ties associated with greater scholarly impact among academic otolaryngologists? Laryngoscope 2017;127:87–94.
44. Baldwin C, Chandran L, Gusic M. Guidelines for evaluating the educational performance of medical school faculty: priming a national conversation. Teach Learn Med 2011;23:285–97.
45. Colleges AoAM. Underrepresented in medicine definition. Available at: https://www.aamc.org/what-we-do/mission-areas/diversity-inclusion/underrepresented-in-medicine#:%7E:text=The%20AAMC%20definition%20of%20underrepresented,

numbers%20in%20the%20general%20population.%22. Accessed September 9, 2020.

46. Tusty M, Flores B, Victor R, et al. The long "race" to diversity in otolaryngology. Otolaryngol Head Neck Surg 2021;164(1):6–8.

47. Ginther DK, Schaffer WT, Schnell J, et al. Race, ethnicity, and NIH research awards. Science 2011;333:1015–9.

48. Check Hayden E. Racial bias continues to haunt NIH grants. Nature 2015;527: 286–7.

49. Fassiotto M, Flores B, Victor R, et al. Rank equity index: measuring parity in the advancement of underrepresented populations in academic medicine. Acad Med 2020;95(12):1844–52.

50. Rodriguez JE, Campbell KM, Mouratidis RW. Where are the rest of us? Improving representation of minority faculty in academic medicine. South Med J 2014;107: 739–44.

51. Epperson M, Gouveia CJ, Tabangin ME, et al. Female representation in otolaryngology leadership roles. Laryngoscope 2020;130:1664–9.

52. Abelson JS, Wong NZ, Symer M, et al. Racial and ethnic disparities in promotion and retention of academic surgeons. Am J Surg 2018;216:678–82.

53. Smith BT, Egro FM, Murphy CP, et al. An evaluation of race disparities in academic plastic surgery. Plast Reconstr Surg 2020;145:268–77.

54. Palepu A, Carr PL, Friedman RH, et al. Specialty choices, compensation, and career satisfaction of underrepresented minority faculty in academic medicine. Acad Med 2000;75:157–60.

55. Sanchez JP, Peters L, Lee-Rey E, et al. Racial and ethnic minority medical students' perceptions of and interest in careers in academic medicine. Acad Med 2013;88:1299–307.

56. Mahoney MR, Wilson E, Odom KL, et al. Minority faculty voices on diversity in academic medicine: perspectives from one school. Acad Med 2008;83:781–6.

57. Pololi L, Cooper LA, Carr P. Race, disadvantage and faculty experiences in academic medicine. J Gen Intern Med 2010;25:1363–9.

58. Richert A, Campbell K, Rodriguez J, et al. ACU workforce column: expanding and supporting the health care workforce. J Health Care Poor Underserved 2013;24:1423–31.

59. Marrast LM, Zallman L, Woolhandler S, et al. Minority physicians' role in the care of underserved patients: diversifying the physician workforce may be key in addressing health disparities. JAMA Intern Med 2014;174:289–91.

60. Hirsch JE. Does the H index have predictive power? Proc Natl Acad Sci U S A 2007;104:19193–8.

61. Bartneck C, Kokkelmans S. Detecting h-index manipulation through self-citation analysis. Scientometrics 2011;87:85–98.

Critical Components of Diversity Initiatives

Brandon I. Esianor, MD[a],*, Nicole Kloosterman, BS[b], Cristina Cabrera-Muffly, MD[c], David J. Brown, MD[d], Kimberly N. Vinson, MD[a]

KEYWORDS

- Diversity • Inclusion • Otolaryngology–head and neck surgery • Recruitment
- Retention • Health equity • Mentorship • Unconscious bias

KEY LEARNING POINTS
AT THE END OF THIS ARTICLE, THE READER WILL:

- Be familiar with the current state of diversity within otolaryngology–head and neck surgery
- Be able to discuss critical components of diversity and inclusion initiatives, including recruitment, retention, mentorship, health equity, and unconscious bias
- Be equipped with a basic framework for creating diversity initiatives

BACKGROUND

The US Census Bureau estimates that minorities currently make up 39.9% of the population, and projects that, by 2045, minorities will collectively become the majority in the United States.[1] Despite the transition of the country to a majority-minority nation, minority groups within medicine continue to be underrepresented. Among active physicians in 2018, 56.2% identified as white, 17.1% identified as Asian, 5.8% identified as Hispanic, and 5.0% identified as black or African American.[2]

The Association of American Medical Colleges (AAMC) emphasizes that increasing diversity within medical school faculty and within academic health centers can reduce health care disparities in the United States.[3–5] As of 2018, the percentage of full-time US medical school faculty is 3.6% black or African American and 5.5% Hispanic, Latino, or of Spanish origin.[2] Both the rapidly evolving composition of the American

[a] Department of Otolaryngology–Head and Neck Surgery, Vanderbilt University Medical Center, 1215 21st Avenue South Suite 7209, Nashville, TN 37232, USA; [b] Vanderbilt University Medical Center, 1215 21st Avenue South Suite 7209, Nashville, TN 37232, USA; [c] Department of Otolaryngology–Head and Neck Surgery, University of Colorado School of Medicine, 12631 E 17th Avenue, Aurora, CO 80045, USA; [d] Department of Otolaryngology–Head and Neck Surgery, Michigan Medicine, 1540 E Hospital Drive, Ann Arbor, MI 48109, USA
* Corresponding author.
E-mail address: Brandon.Esianor@vumc.org

Otolaryngol Clin N Am 54 (2021) 665–674
https://doi.org/10.1016/j.otc.2021.02.007
0030-6665/21/© 2021 Elsevier Inc. All rights reserved.

population and wide-ranging positive implications of improving diversity in the health care workforce necessitate that the diversity of the public is reflected within medicine.

Diversity Trends Within Otolaryngology

Otolaryngology–head and neck surgery (OHNS) has previously been identified as a specialty in the lower tier with regard to minority representation.[6] Approximately 2.4% of actively practicing otolaryngologists in the United States are black, and 3.5% are Hispanic,[2] compared with 12.7% and 16.7% of the total population, respectively.[7] Approximately 1702 (17.68%) women and 7927 (82.32%) men practice OHNS as of 2018.[2]

OHNS-specific data from the Electronic Residency Application Service (ERAS) over the past 5 years (2016–2020) show an increase in the total number of residency applicants from 570 in 2016 to 736 in 2020.[8] The percentage of underrepresented minority (URM) applicants, defined as individuals whose racial and ethnic background is underrepresented in the medical profession relative to their numbers in the general population,[9] within this time period has ranged from 10.3% to 16.7%.[8] The number of applicants from individual minority groups from year to year does not show an identifiable trend over the past 4 years. Nieblas-Bedolla and colleagues[10] analyzed the percentage of matriculants to US surgical subspecialties from 2010 to 2018 and found that OHNS had the lowest mean percentage of matriculants underrepresented in medicine at 8.5%. Schwartz and colleagues[11] conducted a study that investigated the evolution of racial, ethnic, and gender diversity within OHNS surgery residency programs from 1975 to 2010. They found that African Americans and American Indian/Alaskan Natives had nonsignificant annual growth rates, Hispanic Americans had significant increases but at half the growth rate of the Hispanic American population, and women and Asian Americans both had statistically significant growth trends during the study period.[11] A subsequent study in 2016 by Ukatu and colleagues[12] revealed there had not been a significant increase in diversity based on race, ethnicity, or sex since 2010.

The proportions of black and Latino OHNS applicants (7.1% and 6.4% respectively) is similar to representation in medical schools (6.1%, 9.4%); however, a significant decrease occurs when considering the number matching into a residency program (2.3%, 6.2%).[13] Truesdale and colleagues[13] highlighted the "leaky pipeline" within academic OHNS as it pertains to black and Hispanic persons. Along the medical education continuum there is a progressive decline in this population's involvement from medical students, to residency applicants, OHNS residents, assistant professors, associate professors, and to full professors. Strikingly, what begins with a 13% black and 18% Hispanic national population results in 1.7% black and 4.1% Hispanic full professors in OHNS.[13] These findings highlight a systemic issue where lack of racial, ethnic, and gender diversity is exacerbated throughout the career pathway within OHNS.

DISCUSSION

The need for continued improvements in diversity and inclusion within OHNS is becoming increasingly urgent. Through a comprehensive and intentional commitment to diversify the field, clinicians can improve disparities and ensure that the future workforce is representative of society. The state of diversity and inclusion initiatives within OHNS has been described by Smith and colleagues.[14] Of the 99 programs analyzed in that study, 19% had program-specific diversity and inclusion initiatives, 9% had availability of outside resources/funding to women or URMs, 2% had institutional or program-specific benchmarks, and 8% had mentorship or sponsorship programs for women and URMs on program Web sites.

This article augments diversity within OHNS by highlighting key initiatives and programs geared toward recruitment, visibility, retention, unconscious bias, and health equity.

RECRUITMENT OF UNDERREPRESENTED MINORITIES

Expansion of diverse representation within OHNS begins early in the pipeline with recruitment of URMs into medical schools. Various diversity strategies have been highlighted in the undergraduate medical education admissions process, including the creation of a visible mission statement that speaks to diversity enhancement, increasing size and diversity of faculty reviewers, adopting a holistic review, blinding interviewers to academic metrics after an evidence-based cutoff, establishing implicit bias training, and removal of photographs from files when discussing applicants.[15] In addition to stating that programs value diversity during the interview day, the selection committee needs to be as diverse as possible because homogeneous committees do not give URM applicants a sense of belonging.

Holistic review places an emphasis on the whole applicant and deemphasizes traditional quantitative measures used for evaluation.[16] The approach highlights a combination of an individual's background, experiences, attributes, and academic merit. Metrics that loosely correlate with resident success are often used as evaluation strategies because they are easily definable and quantifiable, but they may fail to consider personal characteristics and a variety of educational pathways that would increase consideration for URM applicants. Although there has been a major shift toward this in undergraduate medical education, graduate medical education has been much slower in adopting this process. Several suggestions have been made to facilitate the holistic review process in graduate medical education, including adding a section on family background and disadvantaged status, as well as the incorporation of a section within the ERAS application on noncognitive attributes to represent the applicant.[17]

Residency programs should clearly define ideal characteristics and traits they seek in prospective residents to identify individuals who compliment their department. Examples may include distance traveled, resilience, perseverance, diligence, grit, and working hard. Factors that URM applicants consider when ranking a residency program include diversity of the faculty and residents, a sense of belonging/community, affirming commitment to diversity, serving patients of similar backgrounds, programs with community outreach, and being supported and mentored.

Once matriculated into medical school, early exposure and perceived commitment to OHNS have been noted as crucial components for matriculation.[18] Exposure to OHNS may be particularly limited for students attending schools without an OHNS department or clerkship rotation. Enjoyment of a medical school clerkship was the strongest factor influencing career choice among otolaryngologists of African American or African descent.[19] Effort must be made to increase these opportunities across institutions. Importantly, a previous report on diversity in OHNS found that matriculation of a URM into the program was more likely to occur if there was a minority faculty member in the program.[6] Minority advocacy during the interview process plays an important role in the recruitment of minority residents and can have an impact regardless of the demographic background of the interviewer. As the specialty continues to diversify, an active approach to near-peer mentorship (ie, residents to medical students, junior faculty to residents, and so forth) has the potential to create exponential growth in representation at various levels. Successful minority mentored clerkship initiatives have resulted in increased interest in applying to OHNS residency programs and academic medicine, and expanded research opportunities for involved students.[20] Meaningful experiences and sustained professional support can also create more qualified and interested URM candidates.[21]

OHNS residency program participation in national conferences that cater to URM medical students, such as the Student National Medical Association Annual Medical Education Conference, presents a great opportunity for recruitment efforts. The use of virtual platforms can also prove to be a powerful recruitment tool. In June 2020, 2 URM Vanderbilt OHNS residents hosted a virtual introduction to OHNS session for URM medical students with a focus on increasing exposure to the specialty. The event was a collaboration with other URM residents from programs across the country and attracted roughly 120 URM students. Virtual platforms have led to the creation of new organizations, such as The Black Otolaryngologist Network, geared toward improving URM exposure and education to OHNS across the medical education continuum. The Barnes Society and Society of University Otolaryngologists have established mentorship programs for college and medical students and regularly attend the national and regional Student National Medical Association meetings to expose URM medical students to otolaryngology through hands-on simulation.

FACULTY RETENTION IN ACADEMIA

The presence of URM faculty and leadership can have a significant impact on subsequent generations' pursuit of OHNS, as well as career paths and academic positions. Lett and colleagues[4] specifically evaluated racial and ethnic representation in academic medicine from 1990 to 2016 and found that there were significant trends toward greater underrepresentation for racial minorities in assistant and associate professors within OHNS. Women tended to predominate in the lower ranks of the field's academic ladder, with only 18.4% serving as directors and 5% serving as chairs.[4] These figures make minority faculty retention a critical component in fixing the leaky pipeline within this surgical subspecialty.

Programs with success in increasing retention have included development workshops, mentoring programs, and professional development projects specific to URM junior faculty.[22] Other sources cite strong evidence that faculty development programs and mentoring programs increase retention, productivity, and promotions for URM faculty.[23] Importantly, successful mentorship can occur irrespective of a senior-level faculty's background, ethnicity, or specialty. So long as they have the opportunity to support earlier-career URM otolaryngologists, their advocacy encourages opportunity enhancement.

For women considering surgical careers, inadequate role models and mentorship, as well as concerns about work-life balance and childbearing have been cited as factors affecting fit into a specialty.[24] Women in leadership also have to consider wage gaps[25] and additional household responsibilities compared with their male counterparts.[26] The importance of shared experiences and support helps to retain critical diverse faculty members within academic settings and has the capacity to improve diversity throughout other components of the pipeline as well.

The Johns Hopkins OHNS Department implemented a 10-year diversity initiative from 2004 to 2014 focused on creating a climate of diversity, aggressive recruitment, parity of salary, mentorship, and expansion of the pipeline for minorities and women that resulted in increased representation within their department.[20,27] During the study period, they appreciated an increase in the percentage of women clinical faculty from

5.8% to 23.7%, an increase in URM faculty from 2 to 4, and the promotion of 1 URM faculty to full professor. This initiative highlights the significant impact a proactive diversity initiative can have on representation within a department.

HEALTH EQUITY

Health equity is the absence of unfair and avoidable, or remediable, differences in health among population groups.[28] Although not a common focus in OHNS, a variety of social determinants of health act as factors that influence health inequities within the field. Multiple major otolaryngologic diseases disproportionately affect specific racial and ethnic minority groups.[29] Underserved populations are less frequently diagnosed with common otolaryngologic disorders but are more likely to present with advanced forms of the disease.[30] These findings may indicate a lack of engagement with the health care system, limited access to high-quality health care, or other cultural and socioeconomic barriers that affect risk factors. Despite the importance of these factors in prognosis and in care, research and clinical investigation within the field does not emphasize these determinants of health. Solutions require a multifaceted approach, and institutions with increased physician diversity have higher levels of health disparity and public health research, promote training in cultural competency, and provide mentorship and health policy leadership.[3,4,31]

The importance of diversity in the medical workforce is well established and holds important implications for the physician-patient relationship within OHNS. An example of this is seen within the incidence and survival rates of head and neck cancers between African American and white patients. African Americans have a higher incidence and lower 5-year survival rates compared with their white counterparts, which has been attributed to multiple factors, including a "sense of mistrust that is seen in the African American population."[31] It has been shown that minority patients are more satisfied with racial or ethnically concordant care because of improved communication, resulting in greater health care use and improved health outcomes.[32,33] Minority patients are also more likely to participate in research if members of the team are also of minority groups.[34] Several studies have also shown that URM physicians are more likely to care for underserved populations.[4] Increased diversity within a clinical setting is just 1 step toward alleviating deep-rooted fears and mistrust toward the health care system among marginalized communities. Without focused and intentional efforts to increase diversity in OHNS, there will continue to be a narrowed scope through which patient care and research is conducted, which ultimately serves to widen health disparities across different populations.

UNCONSCIOUS BIAS

Unconscious bias describes prejudice or unsupported judgments in favor of or against one thing, person, or group compared with another, in a way that is usually considered unfair.[35] As both the country and the medical workforce becomes more diverse, institutional changes require a cultural shift toward increased inclusivity. Unconscious bias training is effective for increasing awareness of implicit bias and discrimination, but does not actually reduce biases and has shown limited evidence of behavior change.[36] Training programs implemented in isolation, without other thoughtful programming, may paradoxically reduce diversity metrics, worsening behavior toward minority colleagues, and create illusions of fairness that marginalize the experience of those undergoing discrimination.[37] Considering the mixed impact of isolated bias training, incorporation of ally and bystander training may provide an action-oriented approach that encourages people of all identities to speak out against bias and racism. Although it is not possible to eradicate bias completely, addressing systems and environments in which bias and stereotypes take place can prevent discrimination practices.

STRATEGIC APPROACH TO CREATING DIVERSITY INITIATIVES
Identify Stakeholders and Develop Your Team

Diversity and inclusion initiatives stand to benefit countless aspects within the health care system. Involvement of leadership early in the design process can increase buy-in, ease implementation, and increase sustainability of interventions.[38] Key personnel in a department diversity committee/section may include the program chair, program director, medical student director, research director, faculty diversity champions, residents, and medical students. It is imperative to create a community of diverse allies that includes all demographics, because minority faculty often shoulder a disproportionate responsibility to promote diversity efforts. Inclusion of the ideas and principles of those most affected by the lack of diversity is important in facilitating tailored and expansive reform. Furthermore, voices from various backgrounds must be heard during discussions in order for shared decision making to occur. It is important to welcome unconventional thinking and protect against retaliation in an effort to channel unique insights into meaningful organizational change.[39] If available, consultation with an institutional diversity and inclusion office may prove to be an invaluable resource.

Reflecting on the Past, Analyzing the Present, Preparing for the Future

The term antiracism describes the practice of examining and subtracting the harmful processes within a system in a manner that is active rather than being viewed as new information to learn passively.[40] At an institutional level, there must be synchrony between the statements made about diversity and inclusion and the specific, actionable goals, practices, and initiatives that follow. The case for a diverse health care workforce has been made and repeated calls for an increase in gender, racial, and ethnic diversity within this field require an answer. Institutions must first know what their workforce and patients look like and be able to identify inequities based on demographics. The creation of needs assessments and focus groups can create better understanding within individual OHNS programs of current concerns and help inform future initiatives that make the field more attractive to women and URM applicants. When preparing for the future, it is important to identify how a diverse, equitable, and inclusive workforce can aid in achieving a program's mission and setting specific goals that support this. Being proactive in creating diversity and inclusion strategies is more likely to create a more innovative and compassionate team as opposed to a reactionary response developed to meet diversity and inclusion metrics.

Implementation and Continuous Quality Improvement

Initiatives begin as an action plan that sets realistic goals, contains a specific time frame, highlights action items, and outlines responsible parties for executing a plan.[41] Plans containing readily achievable elements help to build momentum for the overall initiative. The creation of programs to address the diversity gap within OHNS is critical but must be followed by formal auditing and evaluation. Viewing initiatives as fluid, longitudinal commitments rather than static, short-term investments provides opportunities to review and evolve curricula to better meet benchmarks in diversity and inclusion. Interinstitutional collaboration and transparency in initiatives is helpful for idea sharing, decreasing redundancy, and improving efficacy. OHNS is not alone in its push toward broadening its workforce because other surgical subspecialties share similar hurdles and may provide fresh perspectives for program designs and implementation. The review of previous studies and programs outside of OHNS and tracking national trends in diversity within OHNS on a yearly basis will be important for analyzing not only institutional success but also national efforts as well.

Visibility of diversity, equity, and inclusion efforts is just as important as the initiatives themselves: it engages and empowers stakeholders and promotes consistency and accountability in goals. The creation of diversity and inclusion goals that align with each individual department's mission and vision provides clear communication about the commitment to fostering diversity within an institution. For instance, in 2014, Texas A&M Health Science Center College of Medicine established a list of goals in pursuit of their diversity mission with detailed initiatives to support those goals.[42] Transparency in goal setting, data collection, evaluation of change over time, and comparison with other institutions increases accountability around diversity issues.[43] Accountability structures through a diversity officer or task force that monitor this progress can encourage improvements in representation.[44]

SUMMARY

Historically, OHNS has displayed low racial, ethnic, and gender representation. Although many institutions have begun to answer the call to action toward increasing diversity and inclusion within the specialty, there remains much work to be done. There is no single solution to solve the challenges of diversity in OHNS and medicine as a whole. Diversity must become a critical priority within OHNS departments, and a proactive and intentional approach must be adopted to maximize outcomes. Using evidence-based practices, similar to the approach in clinical settings, and expanding on them, can fuel meaningful change. Organizational context matters, and it is important to factor this in when creating initiatives specific to an institution. Ongoing establishment of diversity benchmarks and goals can help continue to widen the welcome of the specialty to those who are underrepresented on an institutional and national level.

CLINICS CARE POINTS

- An increase in diversity efforts can lead to reduction in health care disparities and improved outcomes for patients of all backgrounds.
- Understanding this history of diversity within otolaryngology allows the creation of recruitment and retention initiatives that make the field more attractive to women and underrepresented minorities.
- Proactive and targeted approaches coupled with continuous quality improvement are essential for the success of diversity initiatives.

CONFLICTS OF INTEREST/FINANCIAL DISCLOSURE

None.

REFERENCES

1. Grieco, Elizabeth M., and Rachel C. Cassidy. Overview of race and hispanic origin: 2000, US Census Bureau, Census 2000 Brief. C2KBR/01-1. www.census.gov/prod/2001pubs/c2kbr01-1.pdf, 2001.

2. Diversity in Medicine: Facts and Figures 2019. AAMC, www.aamc.org/data-reports/workforce/report/diversity-medicine-facts-and-figures-2019.

3. Beech BM, Calles-Escandon J, Hairston KG, et al. Mentoring programs for under-represented minority faculty in academic medical centers: a systematic review of the literature. Acad Med 2013;88(4):541.

4. Lett LA, Orji WU, Sebro R. Declining racial and ethnic representation in clinical academic medicine: a longitudinal study of 16 US medical specialties. PLoS One 2018;13(11):e0207274.

5. Cohen JJ. The consequences of premature abandonment of affirmative action in medical school admissions. JAMA 2003;289(9):1143–9.

6. Newsome H, Faucett EA, Chelius T, et al. Diversity in otolaryngology residency programs: a survey of otolaryngology program directors. Otolaryngol Head Neck Surg 2018;158(6):995–1001.

7. HHS, OMH (U.S.. Department of health and human services, office of minority health). 2017. "Minority health profiles. Accessed December 23,2020. https://www.minorityhealth.hhs.gov/omh/browse.aspx?lvl=2&lvlid=26. Available at:.

8. Association of American Medical Colleges. "ERAS statistics." 2018. Available at: https://www.aamc.org/data-reports/interactive-data/eras-statistics-data. Accessed December 23, 2020.

9. Association of American Medical Colleges. "Underrepresented in medicine definition." 2004. Available at: https://www.aamc.org/what-we-do/diversity-inclusion/underrepresented-in-medicine. Accessed December 23, 2020.

10. Nieblas-Bedolla E, Williams JR, Christophers B, et al. Trends in race/ethnicity among applicants and matriculants to us surgical specialties, 2010-2018. JAMA Netw Open 2020;3(11):e2023509.

11. Schwartz JS, Young M, Velly AM, et al. The evolution of racial, ethnic, and gender diversity in US otolaryngology residency programs. Otolaryngol Head Neck Surg 2013;149(1):71–6.

12. Ukatu CC, Welby Berra L, Wu Q, et al. The state of diversity based on race, ethnicity, and sex in otolaryngology in 2016. Laryngoscope 2020;130(12):E795–800.

13. Truesdale CM, Reginald FB, Michael JB, et al. "Prioritizing diversity in otolaryngology–head and neck surgery: starting a conversation.". Otolaryngol Head Neck Surg 2020. https://doi.org/10.1177/0194599820960722.

14. Smith JB, Alexander GC, Kevin JS, et al. "Diversity in academic otolaryngology: an update and recommendations for moving from words to action.". Ear Nose Throat J 2020. https://doi.org/10.1177/0145561320922633.

15. Capers Q, McDougle L, Clinchot DM. Strategies for achieving diversity through medical school admissions. J Health Care Poor Underserved 2018;29(1):9–18.

16. Hupp JR. Holistic review in residency admissions. J Oral Maxillofac Surg 2020; 78(8):1217–8.

17. Williams C, et al. A call to improve conditions for conducting holistic review in graduate medical education recruitment. MedEdPublish 2019;8.

18. National Resident Matching Program. Data release and research committee. Results of the 2016 NRMP program director survey. National Resident Matching Program, Data Release and Research Committee; 2016.

19. Faucett EA, Newsome H, Chelius T, et al. "African American otolaryngologists: current trends and factors influencing career choice.". Laryngoscope 2020; 130(10):2336–42.

20. Nellis JC, Eisele DW, Francis HW, et al. Impact of a mentored student clerkship on underrepresented minority diversity in otolaryngology–head and neck surgery. Laryngoscope 2016;126(12):2684–8.
21. Thomson WA, Denk JP. Promoting diversity in the medical school pipeline: a national overview. Acad Med 1999;74(4):312–4.
22. Daley S, Wingard DL, Reznik V. "Improving the retention of underrepresented minority faculty in academic medicine.". J Natl Med Assoc 2006;98(9):1435.
23. Rodríguez José, Kendall MC, John PF, et al. "Underrepresented minority faculty in academic medicine: a systematic review of URM faculty development.". Fam Med 2014;46(2):100–4.
24. Epperson M, Gouveia CJ, Tabangin ME, et al. Female representation in otolaryngology leadership roles. Laryngoscope 2020;130(7):1664–9.
25. Grandis JR, Gooding WE, Zamboni BA, et al. "The gender gap in a surgical subspecialty: analysis of career and lifestyle factors.". Arch Otolaryngol Head Neck Surg 2004;130(6):695–702.
26. Ferguson BJ, Grandis JR. "Women in otolaryngology: closing the gender gap.". Curr Opin Otolaryngol Head Neck Surg 2006;14(3):159–63.
27. Lin SY, Francis HW, Minor LB, et al. "Faculty diversity and inclusion program outcomes at an academic otolaryngology department.". Laryngoscope 2016;126(2):352–6.
28. A Conceptual Framework for Action on the Social Determinants of Health. World Health Organization, 13 July. 2010, Aug. 2017, https://www.who.int/sdhconference/resources/ConceptualframeworkforactiononSDH_eng.pdf.
29. Bergmark RW, Sedaghat AR. "Disparities in health in the United States: an overview of the social determinants of health for otolaryngologists.". Laryngoscope Investig Otolaryngol 2017;2(4):187–93.
30. Westerberg BD, Lango MN. "Otolaryngology-related disorders in underserved populations, otolaryngology training and workforce considerations in North America.". Otolaryngol Clin North Am 2018;51(3):685–95.
31. Daraei P, Moore CE. "Racial disparity among the head and neck cancer population.". J Cancer Educ 2015;30(3).546–51.
32. Komaromy M, Grumbach K, Drake M, et al. "The role of black and Hispanic physicians in providing health care for underserved populations.". N Engl J Med 1996;334(20):1305–10.
33. Moy E, Bartman BA. "Physician race and care of minority and medically indigent patients.". JAMA 1995;273(19):1515–20.
34. Hamel LM, Penner LA, Albrecht TL, et al. Barriers to clinical trial enrollment in racial and ethnic minority patients with cancer. Cancer Control 2016;23(4):327–37.
35. Vanderbilt University. "Unconscious Bias". 2020. Available at: https://www.vanderbilt.edu/diversity/unconscious-bias/. Accessed December 23,2020.
36. Atewologun, Doyin, Tinu Cornish, and Fatima Tresh. "Unconscious bias training: An assessment of the evidence for effectiveness." Equality and human rights commission research report series (2018).
37. Kang SK, Kaplan S. "Working toward gender diversity and inclusion in medicine: myths and solutions.". Lancet 2019;393:10171.
38. Allen BJ, Garg K. "Diversity matters in academic radiology: acknowledging and addressing unconscious bias.". J Am Coll Radiol 2016;13(12 Pt A):1426–32.
39. Roscigno, Vincent J. The face of discrimination: how race and gender impact work and home lives. Rowman & Littlefield Publishers; 2007.
40. Gutierrez KJ. "The performance of "antiracism" curricula.". N Engl J Med 2020;383(11):e75.

41. Society for human resource management. "How to develop a diversity, equity and inclusion initiative. 2020. Available at: https://www.shrm.org/resourcesandtools/tools-and-samples/how-to-guides/pages/how-to-develop-a-diversity-and-inclusion-initiative.aspx. Accessed December 23, 2020.

42. Association of American Medical Colleges. "Diversity and Inclusion Strategic Plan: Tools and Templates". 2020. Available at: https://www.aamc.org/services/member-capacity-building/diversity-and-inclusion-strategic-planning-toolkit. Accessed December 23, 2020.

43. Pedula D. "Diversion and inclusion efforts that really work.". Harv Bus Rev 2020.

44. Kalev A, Dobbin F, Kelly E. "Best practices or best guesses? Assessing the efficacy of corporate affirmative action and diversity policies.". Am Sociol Rev 2006; 71(4):589–617.

Moving?

Make sure your subscription moves with you!

To notify us of your new address, find your **Clinics Account Number** (located on your mailing label above your name), and contact customer service at:

Email: journalscustomerservice-usa@elsevier.com

800-654-2452 (subscribers in the U.S. & Canada)
314-447-8871 (subscribers outside of the U.S. & Canada)

Fax number: 314-447-8029

Elsevier Health Sciences Division
Subscription Customer Service
3251 Riverport Lane
Maryland Heights, MO 63043

*To ensure uninterrupted delivery of your subscription, please notify us at least 4 weeks in advance of move.